Refined by Fire

A Teen's Journey Through Cancer and Faith

REFINED BY FIRE

A Teen's Journey Through Cancer and Faith

Christian Englert

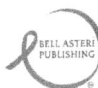

BELL ASTERI
PUBLISHING

Refined by Fire, *A Teen's Journey Through Cancer and Faith*
Copyright ©2025 by Christian Englert
Book cover design copyright ©2025 by Estella Patrick

Author: Christian Englert
Cover Art by Estella Patrick
Foreword by Dr. Joseph F. Matos

Published by Bell Asteri Publishing & Enterprises, LLC
209 West 2nd Street #177
Fort Worth TX 76102
www.bellasteri.com

Published in the United States of America

ISBN: 978-1-957604-62-6 (hardback)
ISBN: 978-1-957604-63-3 (paperback)
ISBN: 978-1-957604-64-0 (electronic book)

WHAT OTHERS ARE SAYING

"It brings me great joy to see Christian's story being shared with the world! There is nothing quite like someone's story to give you hope in those difficult and uncertain moments in life. How do you respond when life doesn't go the way you planned it? What do you do when God's does not make sense and leaves you asking the question, 'Why?' I believe Christian's story will inspire many to courageously trust God in those moments, move forward in faith, and witness Jesus do something next in their life that is only possible through him!"

Derric Bonnot
Executive Worship Pastor
Fellowship Church Dallas

"Though familiar with much of the story, I found myself amazed at the honesty and transparency of Christian's writing. At times, the reader will feel as if he is walking alongside Christian, his family, church community, and the medical team who are all part of this story. The reader will laugh, cry, and be entranced by the narrative. At its conclusion, you will want to stand up and cheer. This is a tremendous story of faith, family, community, courage, and both medical and spiritual miracles. If you or someone you know is going through a crisis of faith or an unexpected and overwhelming physical or medical challenge, this book is for you. Undoubtedly, Christian and his family asked the question *Why us?* I am pleased to say that the publication of this book is one answer to that penetrating question."

Michael E. Williams, Sr.
Senior Professor of History
Dallas Baptist University

"How do you respond when life hits you out of nowhere? Do you freeze, flee, or fight? Many people become paralyzed with fright. Others run out of fear. Some, though, rely on their faith and fight with everything they have. These stories – the stories of relying on faith and overcoming insurmountable odds – are the stories that inspire us. This is Christian's story.

In *Refined by Fire*, Christian unpacks a story that is both frightening and inspiring. The battle he and his family have faced is the kind none of us want to face. Yet, through these pages, he demonstrates what real faith looks like and how it can sustain anyone through the toughest of times. With vulnerability and transparency, this young man shows us all that the fires we face in life are often the very things God uses to teach us to live a life of faith. We will be forever grateful that he and his family trusted us to fight alongside them. And we will never forget the faith he demonstrated in the good times and the bad through his battle."

The Boyd Family

FOREWORD

Dr. Joseph F. Matos
Professor of Biblical Studies
Dallas Baptist University

YouTube Creator: "On Journey with Dr. Joseph Matos"
(youtube.com/@DrJosephFMatos)
Co-founder with Christian: JourneytotheTruth.org

When I met Christian, his life was in crisis - his academic life. When Christian began attending Dallas Baptist University, he was undecided about his major. As a result, he was initially advised by a staff member in the Advising Center. That staff member wisely instructed Christian to take courses in a major he was considering, so he did. Two of the first classes he took in that potential major were Spiritual Formation and Principles of Biblical Interpretation, required courses for Biblical Studies majors.

When Christian declared his major, it was the accelerated Bachelor of Arts in Biblical Studies and Master of Arts in Theological Studies. Upon his declaration, I became his advisor. But he had a problem. The accelerated program at the time identified two specific graduate courses to be shared with the undergraduate major. This avoided repetition of content at both undergrad and graduate levels while saving students six credit hours in the program. The problem, the crisis, for Christian, was that he had already taken those two very courses at the undergraduate level. How could he do the accelerated program after that? He still could do a master's degree, but unless something could be done, he would have to repeat those two courses at the graduate level. What could be done? He had fears about his degree plan.

His academic crisis was nothing compared to the physical and spiritual crises he faced just a few years prior, not to mention the fears that went along with them. In high school, one of his greatest fears became reality - he was diagnosed with brain cancer. That diagnosis led to doubts about his once-strong faith and his belief in the existence of God. The outcome of these parallel crises (Christian calls them trials in his book) would affect his future. Had the second crisis not been resolved, Christian would not have had to worry about his academic crisis, for he might not have selected the accelerated program, even if he did attend DBU. Had the first crisis not been resolved, he would not have attended any school.

By the time I started advising Christian, I had already known he was a cancer survivor. But by the strong faith he possessed and the passion he had (and has) for the Lord, I would never have guessed that he had wrestled so long and hard about his faith. Christian's faith in Jesus Christ is rock solid. I have had the privilege of witnessing Christian's strong faith in action both as his academic advisor and as his professor for four semesters of Greek (a process that will test anyone's faith), Christianity in a Pluralistic World, and Later Life and Letters of Paul. I would learn that it is a faith that came with great struggle. It came as a result of a period in the refiner's fire. You will learn this as well as you read this book.

Christian's story is amazing and the way he tells it will keep you reading. He relates his journey in a gripping way, keeping your attention as you await the next episode in the narrative. As fixated as you will be reading this book, prepare yourself. This is not a simple story of "God healed me and now I believe." This is a true wrestling with deep questions and doubts about God throughout the journey. Along the way, Christian receives "timely" reassurances from unexpected places, in unexpected events, and by unexpected people. He will offer real and deep reflection about the outcome of the journey. Hear him well.

Christian is an amazing young man. He has a great mind. He has endured a lot. He is an overcomer. Through all his struggles physically and spiritually, he has become such a great encouragement to others. He truly is an encourager. He is one of my biggest encouragers. Today, we are no longer advisor/advisee nor professor/student. We are now ministry partners, working together in the areas of discipleship and apologetics. In all of this, he is so affirming of me in my endeavors as a professor and writer. I don't take his encouragement lightly. It is encouragement from the heart. But he is living out what I have long said about his writing this book.

In January 2020, while I was still only his advisor, as he had not yet taken any classes with me, he shared that he was writing a book about his bout with cancer. Even then, he was asking a deep question about prayer and the interpretation of a passage of scripture he was looking to include in the book. The first words I wrote to him before giving a long-winded (and maybe not so helpful) answer was: "I know you will be encouraging a lot of people with what you write." I said that before reading one word of the book. I just knew Christian and therefore I knew the result of his work.

I have now read the completed book, and I stand by those words I wrote five years ago. You will be encouraged by what Christian writes. You might be struggling with doubts. Your trial may not be cancer. As Christian acknowledges in the opening chapter, trials come in different forms. The effects on faith, however, may be the same. His encouragement comes from his experience. He, too, received encouragement along the way.

Finally, recognize that this book is about the journey through dual crises, not just about beating cancer. It is about the process of the refining of faith, the renewal of faith, Christian experienced.

On May 8, 2024, Christian graduated with his accelerated bachelor's and master's degrees after we found a solution to his academic crisis (and he successfully completed all his classes). It involved a timely course change in the graduate program to account for one class and a course substitution to account for the other. On top of that, he minored in History. All of this from a student who was told he likely would not be able to go to college as a result of all the cancer treatment he would endure. More significantly, almost a decade prior, Christian and a team of others took the appropriate and needed steps to help him get through both his physical and spiritual crises. As you read this book about Chrisian's journey, you will be inspired and encouraged as you make your way on your journey or help someone else on theirs.

ACKNOWLEDGMENTS

I am forever grateful to...

My Lord and Savior, Jesus Christ. He is the reason for everything. I dedicate this book, my physical healing, the restoration of my faith, and my ultimate eternity to Him.

My mom, Shanna. You are the epitome of a selfless caregiver. You are one of the closest people to me, and you have walked alongside me through the tears, pain, joy, and gratitude. You have encouraged me at my best and seen me through my worst. You have unconditionally supported this book and encouraged me to trust in the plans God has for us. And as you have now walked through and beaten cancer yourself, you know what that entails.

My dad, Martin. You have shown me what true confidence in God looks like. You have protected our family and provided strength when we needed it most. You support me unconditionally and encourage the person God created me to be. You are the most influential male in my life and have shown me what it looks like to be a man of God.

My sister, Lauren. You are one of my biggest heroes. I have always tried to be a good big brother to you, but I look up to you in more ways than you may know. You are one of the humblest people I know, and you are a constant source of joy in our family. You are a light in our family that will never stop shining.

My grandmother, Mimi. As the matriarch of our family, you have watched over us with great strength and care. You are a fountain of wisdom, and I have always been encouraged to come to you when I need sound advice. Additionally, your investment in my writing ability is unparalleled. No one has influenced it more than you.

My grandfather, Pop. You are the best grandfather I could have ever asked for. I don't think anyone could love his grandkids more than you have loved me, Lauren, Brittany, and Austin. You have been a constant source of encouragement. In many ways, I attribute my love for Scripture and passion for ministry to your influence on me.

My Oma. I praise God for blessing me and Lauren with you as a grandmother. You are one of the strongest women I know. You have passed our German heritage to me, and you are the reason I cherish it so much. You have taught me the importance of family. We lean on each other, and you will always have a special place in my heart.

My extended family. God provided you in a great multitude, but each one of you has had a great impact on my life. In some cases, we are separated by hundreds of miles, but no distance could ever hinder the love and support we have for each other. I love each one of you more than you will ever know.

Ed and Lisa Young, and my entire church family. You have had a resounding influence on my life. You have invested in my relationship with Christ and surrounded my family as we walked through the journey of cancer—twice. I will never forget this.

The Boyd Family. You guys are much more than friends and mentors. You are family. The impact you have had on my faith journey is priceless. Jackson, I consider you a brother and will never forget the countless ways you have shown up when I needed you most.

Dr. Murray, Dr. Honeycutt, Mandy, and the rest of my medical team. There is no doubt in my mind that God used you immensely in the process of my physical healing. Yet, you provided more than knowledge and skill that culminated in success. You have provided prayer and care that is invaluable to my family. We love each of you.

Mrs. Morris and Ms. Bernard. I don't know how I would have gotten through my sophomore year of high school without you. You did not just teach and help me with schoolwork, though. You lifted me up on tough days and prayed for me as the process of cancer treatment ran its course.

Madison Gillespie. You are, without a doubt, the most influential English teacher I have ever had. But you did more than just teach me. When I was trying to adjust back to public school after treatment, you were in my corner and cared for me when I faced new challenges. You encouraged me and constantly invested in my writing ability. I would not be such a passionate writer if not for you.

Dr. Jodi Grimes. Beyond being an incredible English professor, you are a faithful friend and mentor. As I wrote this book, you helped me constantly. When writer's block hit, you were there to help me talk through organizing tough sections. This book came together in large part because of you.

Dr. Mike Williams. You are one of the most influential mentors in my life. As I walked through college, you were there to advise and encourage me in everything that came with it. I love you and consider you to be family.

Dr. Joseph Matos. I can't thank you enough for writing the foreword of this book. I believe you are going to change Christian scholarship in mighty ways. You are much more than a professor and partner in ministry. You have become one of my greatest mentors, and I consider you to be family.

Make-A-Wish®. I cannot thank you enough for the ways you have blessed my family. It is because of this organization that we were able to rejuvenate from the nine-month rollercoaster of cancer treatment. We will never forget the generosity of this organization and continue to tell people about its impact on kids who face life-threatening illnesses.

The vast army of prayer warriors. To all those who visited my family, provided meals for us, encouraged us, and prayed for us as we faced the challenge of cancer, I thank you. And truthfully, no words can express the appreciation that my family and I have for you. We love you.

CHAPTER ONE

Isn't it funny how life throws us a curveball in the middle of a strong at-bat? Both physically and mentally, we might be on a roll. Physically, we are healthier than ever before, filled with energy, and enjoy getting up every day. Mentally, our fears don't control us, our anxiety is low, and our mind is filled with joy.

But then the curveball is thrown. We know how it moves, but it is a hard pitch to hit. And even worse, we don't see it coming. In life, this curveball I am talking about is called a trial.

Trials can be tricky because they come in different shapes and sizes. They may involve challenges such as striving for good grades in school or tackling a frustrating home improvement project. Trials can also take the shape of more significant life events, like the end of a relationship, fighting a disease, or coping with the loss of a loved one.

Trials are not only tricky, but it doesn't take a genius to realize they are also no fun. No one wakes up in the morning and thinks, "Man, I hope I get in a car wreck today!" That would be absurd. In fact, you could argue that humans do the exact opposite. A majority of us tend to run away from suffering in life.

Each person responds to trials differently. Two people could lose a job, but they might react in different ways. Neither will be happy, but depending on who they are, one might see it as an opportunity to grow, while the other might become negative and dwell in the hurt that exists. The two individuals might also take different pathways to overcome the trial. One of them might turn to addiction, while the other might start praying and asking God for help.

Life is full of trials. No matter who you are, how much money you have, or what your worldview is, you will suffer in this life. That is a daunting reality. And I would say that we all wrestle with the reality of suffering at one point or another.

Many of us wrestle with questions like these: *Why do we go through trials? How do we overcome trials? Can any good come from them?*

If you believe in a loving God who cares for each of us individually, it can be confusing to imagine His existence in a world filled with tragedy and pain. Many who believe in God ask, "If there is a loving God who is powerful enough to stop suffering, why does He let us experience it?" This is one of the most difficult questions to answer.

Many people who don't believe in God have arrived at that conclusion because they cannot reconcile the existence of God and pain together. The notion that a loving God could permit His creation to suffer seems absurd.

I can see where they are coming from. The existence of trials troubled me throughout my early life, leading me to spend much time and energy trying to make sense of them. Ultimately, I discovered that navigating through these trials is often necessary to uncover their true purpose. I would have to encounter and journey through the biggest trial I could have imagined to gain some understanding of why we suffer in life.

Life Came Crashing Down

It all started when I was entering my sophomore year of high school. During this season, life appeared great on the outside. I had begun drumming at my church's youth group and was almost at the level where I could play on the worship team at weekend services. I was ready to tackle a new year in school and succeed in every class. I also had formed a good group of friends, and I was looking forward to attending as many high school football games as I could with them.

However, there was a minor physical problem that raised concern: my hand tremors were getting worse. These tremors were not a recent development. They had been present my whole life. My hands had consistently shaken for fifteen years. And it was because of a tremor-filled family history that my pediatrician had diagnosed them as genetic. At the beginning of my sophomore year, though, the tremors got much worse. My hands were getting so shaky that I could barely write.

After months of uncontrollable shaking, we decided that my tremors needed to be reassessed. So, at my annual exam, we asked my pediatrician to take a look at my hands. As before, he felt they were simply genetic, but he also thought it would be a good idea to get a second opinion from a neurologist, so we scheduled an appointment to get the neurologist's perspective.

About a week before meeting with the neurologist, I began to experience a throbbing pain in the back of my head. While this pain was more annoying than anything else, it also scared me. Since I was facing an impending appointment with a neurologist due to a possible problem in my head, I couldn't shake the feeling that something serious might be wrong. My tendency to be a hypochondriac didn't help.

From a young age, I grappled with a fear of brain cancer, influenced by my family's extensive history of various cancers. I watched lymphoma take my granddad's life when I was six years old. He initially defeated the lymphoma, but it came back with a vengeance, and it was hard to process. Despite my young age, I was so concerned for my grandfather that one day, I went over to my grandma's house with the mission of curing cancer. She said that I was all dressed up. I wanted to use her computer for research, convinced I could discover a way to heal my grandfather. You might say this was a tall task for a six-year-old.

The impact of facing cancer at a young age created an ongoing fear of the disease. I worried that I would have cancer one day, and I always believed that brain cancer was the worst. I reasoned that since the brain plays such a crucial role in the body, cancer in that region felt like an inevitable death sentence.

When I began experiencing that pain in the back of my head, I was gripped with fear. I could not get brain cancer out of my mind, and I began to have dreams about a doctor breaking the news that cancer was in my brain. I tried to tell myself I had nothing to worry about, but the fear never left. It felt like brain cancer was chasing me down.

Appointment day arrived. My mom picked me up from school early, and we headed to the clinic to see the neurologist. Externally, I tried to mask my anxiety, but internally, I was struggling. There was some excitement about getting out of school early, but deep down, I was preparing myself for when the neurologist told us that I had brain cancer. Now, I realize how dramatic that was, especially because he couldn't see inside my brain with magical powers. Nevertheless, the fears were there.

We arrived at the doctor's office, and the appointment began. It lasted about an hour. My neurologist conducted some simple tests, which did not seem to raise much concern in his mind. He then spent a significant amount of time explaining how common hand tremors are and how many people live normal lives with them. Additionally, he provided me with some strategies to use when writing and some encouraging remarks to keep in mind when people noticed that I had hand tremors.

He wanted to conduct a couple more tests before letting us go. During one of the tests, he noticed a slight twitch in my trunk, which seemed slightly abnormal. After completing the test, he said,

"I do think the hand tremors are genetic, but let's have an MRI just to make sure." This was a calming yet scary statement. It was calming because, after all the tests, he still believed there was nothing wrong. But it was scary because he wanted me to get an MRI. He assured us that it was just a precaution, but fear of the MRI had already started to overwhelm me.

Over the next week, I went through each day as calmly as possible. I tried to replace my anxiety with schoolwork, drumming, and anything else that freed me from having to think about the results of the upcoming MRI. It wasn't easy, though. I was terrified about what my doctors would find in the scan. To make matters worse, I concealed my anxiety about the MRI from my parents and family. I didn't want to stir up a commotion. No one else in my family was apprehensive about this at all. My parents even almost canceled the MRI, but in a way I hadn't yet realized, I would be glad they ultimately decided to proceed with it.

MRI day arrived, and my anxiety surged intensely. Once more, I attempted to concentrate on school and push my fear aside, but it was futile. My mom believed I was anxious due to the unfamiliar medical test I was about to undergo. However, that wasn't the true reason for my nerves.

I checked out of school early (this time, there was no excitement about missing school) and headed to the MRI facility. On the way, my mom repeatedly assured me that the MRI would be over soon and we would move on with life. I wanted to believe that so badly.

We arrived and checked in. My mom was busy filling out a mountain of paperwork while I was going nuts on the inside.

Shortly after, an MRI technician came out to guide us back for the scan.

As we walked back, the technician explained that MRIs are loud and lengthy. To relieve some of the noise and monotony, though, they would give me headphones that could play music from my phone.

This did not ease my anxiety. Loud, startling noises have been a fear of mine since I was little. The fact that I was about to endure 45 minutes of them was not amusing. My anxiety was escalating, but there was no turning back.

Soon, I entered the room and lay down on a movable bed positioned outside the machine. The technician adjusted my position and placed a cage-like device over my head. It had a mirror allowing me to see the front of the room and the window behind which she would be working. Once she had completed the setup, she rolled my bed back into the tube. The loud noises started, but the headphones canceled out the sound pretty well. My playlist also diverted my focus, and to this day, I can remember most of the songs I was listening to. This indicates just how much I was trying to focus on them during the MRI rather than my fear.

As the scan progressed, I tried to focus my attention on the music instead of the underlying fear about the results.

At one point, the MRI machine stopped making noise, and the technician informed me through the headphones that she would be coming in to help me out of the machine. I assumed this meant my scan was complete, and I was filled with eagerness to get off the table. However, after rolling me out of the machine, she told my mom and me that the doctor wanted to get a few more images of my brain. He also wanted to administer contrast to enhance the clarity of the pictures. The technician inserted an IV in my arm, and we engaged in some small talk to help pass the time.

Once she finished setting up the IV, she rolled me back into the tube, and we proceeded with the additional tests. About five minutes into the next set of pictures, the technician returned and waved my mom out of the room.

I watched all of this happen, and it made my heart race. "Brain tumor" was the only thought that crossed my mind, and I couldn't stay still. My mind raced and raced until I saw Mom enter the room again as if nothing was wrong. My heartbeat slowed down, and the word "tumor" began to fade from my mind.

A few minutes later, the MRI ended, and the technician came in and rolled me out of the tube. I was so glad to be done. I ran into the other room to grab my phone from the technician's desk, eager to leave as quickly as possible. In addition to my desire to distance myself from the MRI machine, I had a rehearsal for my youth group that evening and was running slightly behind schedule. However, before I could reach my phone, my mom called me over to join her in the hallway.

My mom and I walked into the hallway where the lockers were located. After taking a moment to collect her thoughts, she informed me that I wouldn't be able to attend rehearsal that night. This confused me because we still had plenty of time to make it before rehearsal ended.

As we approached the lockers, I sat down, and she said, "It

seems that they have found an abnormality in your brain."

My heart sank. I immediately thought, "*CANCER*!" But I did have a sliver of hope that because my mom mentioned "abnormality", it could signify something other than a "tumor".

So, I asked, "What does that mean?"

Before she even answered, I knew what she had originally meant by "abnormality." Her body language said it all. I don't know if I can recall another time in my life when I have seen the same look of worry on my mom's face. All I could conclude was that it had to be a tumor.

She paused and then confirmed, "It seems that they have found a mass in your brain, and we need to head to the hospital right away."

When she informed me that a mass had been discovered and we needed to rush to the hospital's emergency room, I felt overwhelmed by trauma. Although I didn't know the details about the mass in my brain, I sensed that my life was at stake at that moment.

I started to hyperventilate uncontrollably, and my heart raced rapidly. My mom took my hands and said, "Christian. Right now, we have to put our complete faith in God. We don't have any answers. But God does because He was in this moment before you were born, and He is not surprised by this." She then started to pray and asked God to take control and provide peace in the unknown. I felt trapped in a hole that was impossible to get out of. The only one who had the power to rescue in this situation was God, and yet, putting faith in Him seemed impossible.

CHAPTER TWO

It may seem understandable that I struggled to put faith in God while I was standing in the hallway. There was a lot to process during that moment. When faced with tough news, it isn't always easy to trust the God we believe in. Yet, there was another factor that hindered my ability to put faith in the Lord.

An Underlying Problem

Since I was a child, faith has been an important part of my life. Family members have shared that I began asking them profound questions about God at a surprisingly young age, often leaving them unable to answer. One of my grandmother's cherished memories is when, at just three years old, I requested my grandfather to explain what a sign from God meant while he tucked me into bed. But my interest in Jesus extended beyond just family interactions.

In elementary school, while my friends wanted to talk about the hottest toys and best sports teams, I often shifted the conversation to Jesus. These attempts were rarely successful, as eight-year-olds are not typically captivated by the notion that humanity has sinned and needs to repent to Jesus. Nevertheless, I pressed on and told everyone about my savior.

As I transitioned into middle school, my conversations with others about Jesus became more appropriate. Along the way, I met not only fellow believers in Jesus but also individuals who believed in different gods and some who didn't believe in God at all. Those who held differing views on religion frequently posed questions about Jesus, and I was generally able to respond. Even when I did not have an answer, though, I could consult a pastor at church and bring their explanation back to school with me. Different beliefs and challenges were not enough to rock my faith.

Upon entering high school, I found that these questions and challenges became increasingly difficult to refute. It even got to the point where I could not answer the questions I received from non-believers. Some of these pertained to the origin of the world's existence, others to the validity of Jesus' resurrection. I felt trapped, which led to my own doubts emerging. I attempted to suppress them and forget about them, but they lingered and refused to disappear.

My questions eventually morphed into doubts about God. As months passed, these doubts only continued to grow and become more powerful. I started to wonder if I believed in the right God or if God existed at all.

I didn't realize that everyone experiences doubt and that questions and doubts are common. Even leaders in the Bible experienced these things. Moses, whom God appointed as the leader of His people, suffered from the effects of doubt. Yet, I did not realize this, and I began to think I wasn't "Christian enough" to be a follower of Jesus... if He was real.

I was also afraid of the reaction I would get from others. This included my parents, who had invested so much in me and were proud of my faith in God. I thought that if I shared what I was experiencing, their response would be one of worry and disappointment. The thought of disappointing my parents and peers was enough to keep me silent, so I told nobody about my doubt in Jesus.

I was discouraged in my faith and did not know what to do. After months of silently wrestling with my doubts and searching for answers alone, I ultimately decided to stop looking. Just weeks before my appointment with my pediatrician, I had decided to move on with life and hoped that my convictions would resolve themselves. I hoped that maybe focusing on the joys of playing drums and hanging out with friends would be enough to starve my doubts and make them go away. I was wrong.

The Resilience of Doubt

As we continued through the process of getting to the MRI, my doubt was fed by the fear and anxiety that continued to pile on. It felt like a 100-pound weight was on my chest. My mom thought I was just nervous about the MRI experience, but it was much deeper than that. I was being torn apart by doubt and the sudden terror caused by the overwhelming fear of having a brain tumor. This drove me further away from God.

I remember one night when I lay in bed, overwhelmed by anxiety and unable to sleep. Out of desperation, I prayed with anger toward the God I doubted. I told Him there was no way He would let me face something as terrible as a brain tumor. How ridiculous, right? Here I was, telling the God of all creation what was going to happen.

Job 21:22 says, *"Can anyone teach knowledge to God since he judges even the highest?"*

I believe this is how God responded to me at that moment. I was so fearful of something that hadn't even happened that I tried to judge the God I was doubting. And I told Him He could not allow something as bad as a brain tumor to happen to me. But we cannot dictate to God how things are going to be. He is the creator and sustainer of everything in existence, and He directs every little thing that happens.

Despite everything, I held onto my anger and desperation. This would not help, though. On the day of the MRI, I experienced the same anxiety that had been haunting me, convinced that the scan would reveal something significant. Although listening to music helped during the procedure, fear remained in my mind.

I had a sliver of hope that nothing would be wrong. However, when the technician took my mom out of the room during the latter part of the scan, my thoughts quickly shifted to the worst-case scenario. I knew there was a problem. Yet nothing could have prepared me for the news I was going to hear when I got off the MRI table.

The Impact of Reality

It is hard to describe what it feels like to have your worst fear come true as mine did in that hallway. I guess I could equate it to feeling like someone reaching inside your chest, grabbing your heart, and twisting it around before ripping it out (no wonder I was searching for the ability to breathe). There is also the feeling of being slapped in the face and having the floor ripped from under you at the same time.

Now, you would think that with all the worrying I did before the MRI and the history of fearing brain cancer, I wouldn't be too shocked to hear the news about a mass in my brain. I must admit that a part of me felt as if a brain tumor had chased me down.

That is the power of your worst fear becoming true, though. When the floor was ripped out from under me, I realized that I was no longer dealing with mere doubt—an uncertainty about what might be true. I was facing reality. The things that had been worrying me for the past few weeks were true, and my attempt to escape my doubt failed in the worst way possible.

The Beginning of a Long Journey

The drive to the hospital felt like an eternity. Not only were we trying to find our way there, but we were also making calls to people who needed to know what was going on. Each call became tougher to listen to. Hearing repeatedly that I had a mass in my brain and was being rushed to the hospital did not sit well in my stomach.

One of the most memorable calls we made in the car was to my Aunt Tabi. As soon as she heard, "He has a mass in his brain," she told us she was on her way.

"Don't come yet," replied my mom, "We don't have a lot of details about what is going on, and I am not even sure where we will go beyond the fact that they told us to head to the emergency room."

"OK, whatever," said my aunt, and then she ended the call.

At some point between calls, my mom asked me if there was anyone that I wanted to call. At that moment, I thought about many people. God had put many impactful individuals in my life. However, there was one person I felt truly needed to hear the news more than anyone else.

To this day, that person is one of my best friends in the entire world. I have known Jackson since before we could talk. Throughout our friendship, he has had my back and has wanted the best for my life. This support is mutual. We lift each other in weak moments and have a huge influence on each other.

I said, "I would like to call Jackson."

She responded, "OK. I will call his dad."

The phone began to ring through the car's Bluetooth. I found myself wondering what we would say if his dad picked up.

It wasn't long before we heard "Hello?" on the other end, which was followed with silence. We broke the news to Jackson's father, Mr. Andy, who was at a loss for words. Mr. Andy is another person I have been close to. He has served as an additional father figure in my life, and it broke my heart that we had to deliver such bad news.

Once he composed himself, Mr. Andy led us in a prayer. I can still remember being filled with fear at that moment but resting on the prayerful words he spoke. I will always be thankful for that prayer and the countless others that followed.

The conversation with Mr. Andy was similar to many of the calls we made during that car ride. Almost everyone was at a loss for words, eager to offer assistance, and requested to pray for us. Telling someone you have a brain tumor is almost as hard as receiving the news yourself.

Upon arriving at the hospital, we headed to the emergency waiting room, which was packed with people. The sight of a hospital emergency room was daunting for me. I had been afraid of hospitals my whole life. The presence of sick people in hospitals always filled me with sadness and anxiety for them. But this situation was different. This time, I was the sick person. I didn't have any choice but to confront my fear and embrace the hospital.

As I stood at the entrance of the room for just a few seconds, I observed a variety of situations unfolding. Some kids appeared to be suffering from the flu, while others looked like they had an injury. I started to assess their situations against mine and honestly wished I could have the flu or a broken bone. I will say that comparing yourself to others is a dangerous thing to do. But at that moment, I wanted to be in any other position than the one I was in.

As we entered the emergency room, my mom had no idea who to approach to say, "Yes, my son has a tumor in his brain. Where do we go?"

Eventually, we found a nurse who led us to the right person. Before I knew it, I was in the part of the emergency room where patients were receiving treatment. We got our own spot in the ER, and nurses started to take my height, weight, blood pressure, and every other vital known to man. The gravity of my situation began to set in. It wasn't that I had somehow fallen asleep in that MRI tube and had an intense nightmare. I was truly a patient requiring urgent care.

My dad arrived at the hospital and found our room. You could see his emotions all over his face. He was experiencing every emotion that had consumed my mom and me for the last couple of hours. We were confused, uncertain about what the evening would bring. To make matters worse, the hospital staff seemed just as unsure.

Shortly after, a nurse came in and informed us that I would be relocated to another room in the ER. Once I was transferred, a new team of nurses started asking us the same series of questions regarding our reason for visiting the hospital. We recounted everything that had happened up to that moment, and they assured us that a doctor would arrive shortly. The emotions continued to rise for my parents and me, and then suddenly, the door flew open...

Standing in the entryway was my aunt. At first, I was confused, but then I remembered the phone conversation she had with my mom while we were on our way to the hospital. I knew by the way she said, "OK, whatever," that she was going to disobey my mom's wishes.

My aunt is someone who will do whatever she puts her mind to, regardless of the obstacles. So, the fact that she found my room was child's play. She can also lighten the mood in any room, and she has always been able to put a smile on my face.

Although my mom preferred that my aunt not come until we had more details, her presence turned out to be a true blessing. My dad had recently arrived at the hospital, and we needed someone to comfort us. She managed to keep a smile on my face while the nurses attended to me. She even pulled a taser out of her purse and asked me if she should make it go off to see how my mom would react. This sparked great laughter and helped distract me from the overwhelming situation that was playing out.

As I lay in bed, my mom began receiving messages from all sorts of people. Each text included a mention of prayer. I was blown away that within just an hour, so many people were already offering their support during a storm they knew little about. The flow of messages continued without pause, and all I could hear from my bed was the constant sound of "buzz... buzz... buzz..."

My mom turned to me and said, "I'm amazed at all the texts we

19

are getting."

I said, "Yeah! Has Derric (my church's head worship leader) texted?"

"No, he probably doesn't even know. You have to remember that it hasn't been that long since the MRI ended. So, I don't know who all has heard about our situation," she said. Shortly after, though, I heard her say, "Wow!" She turned to me, phone in hand, and said, "Guess who just texted?"

She placed her phone in front of me, revealing a text from Derric on the screen. As my mom began to read the message aloud, she became emotional, moved by the comforting and encouraging words he had shared.

She finished reading and asked (sarcastically), "Is there anyone else you would like to hear from?"

I laughed and said, "Yeah, pastor Ed!" Pastor Ed is my senior pastor. I wasn't expecting us to receive a text from him or his family.

But to our amazement, within minutes, "buzz..."

My mom looked at me in shock. On her phone was a message from our senior pastor's wife that stated she and Pastor Ed were in prayer.

The Impact of Support

Our daunting journey, facing whatever the tumor had in store, was just starting. However, support immediately appeared along our path.

As we were settling into the emergency room, God used my aunt. With so much happening around us, anxiety gripped our hearts. Yet, I truly believe that God used her to bring us laughter. To this day, I'm not sure how she managed to enter the emergency room and locate us. Nevertheless, my aunt provided immense comfort during a challenging time.

When I think back to the early texts and prayers we received in that hospital room, I am amazed at how God worked through them. My parents and I were facing a trial for which we were completely unprepared. We all felt lost, confused, sad, and scared. With no control over the situation, we were in desperate need of support.

The texts we received provided more than just support. Above all, hearing from our loved ones brought us comfort. Reflecting on that time, I genuinely believe that God used each message as a guiding hand to hold us steady while everything felt like it was spiraling out of control.

Additionally, the texts reassured us that even though we had only just embarked on a challenging journey with no clear end in sight, we were not alone. Any military leader will affirm that it's more advantageous to enter battle with a vast army rather than a few soldiers. The collective voices of many reminded us that, regardless of what addressing the mass in my brain involved, we were advancing into battle with a full army behind us. This provided strength, security, and motivation in my heart.

You may be curious about how the texts impacted my faith during that time. I found it peculiar that certain people I had hoped would reach out did so with messages of encouragement and prayer. This was particularly surprising since we hadn't informed them about the tumor ourselves. While news can spread like wildfire, there were other factors at play as well.

Although we regarded Derric as a spiritual leader in our lives, we didn't communicate with him regularly. We hadn't shared anything on social media, and only a handful of people were aware of the situation. Additionally, Derric served as the lead worship leader at a large church, making him extremely busy. The chances of him hearing about my predicament seemed slim. It was a similar dynamic with Pastors Ed and Lisa.

The timing of each text was perfect. I sensed a deeper meaning behind those messages. My childhood experiences of worshiping and sharing Jesus led me to believe it was God reaching out. But my doubts were so overwhelming that I struggled to recognize a loving God permitting the trials I was facing. When I attempted to trust Him in that moment, I wasn't able to do so sincerely. This is something I would wrestle with for the next few months.

The Last Night

After speaking with the doctor, my parents learned that my hydrocephalus was very severe, requiring my transfer from the ER to the ICU. This emphasized the gravity of an already critical situation. The medical team was unsure about the exact course of action to take. I had no one to turn to for an answer. All we knew was that I was in a dire situation, which might lead to a massive surgery and, possibly, death.

Shortly after the doctor informed us about the ICU, the hospital staff arrived to relocate my bed. We arrived at my corner of the intensive care unit, where nurses swarmed my bed again. They asked me questions, took my vitals, and inserted a needle into my arm.

Soon after, a doctor entered and took my parents aside. I assumed he was there to discuss a plan for the next steps.

The nurses continued to take tests and tried to explain what was going on. In the waning hours, it became increasingly likely that I would undergo brain surgery. I was apprehensive because I had never been through any surgery, and now a surgeon was going to be digging around in my head.

To better understand what to expect, I bombarded them with numerous questions about the surgery. I planned to prepare myself as thoroughly as possible for the upcoming procedure.

Upon concluding their discussion with the ICU doctor, my parents returned to the room and informed me that I was scheduled for surgery the following morning. My surgeon would meet with us beforehand to provide details about the procedure. They noted that the doctor wasn't aware of the specific details of the surgery, but he anticipated that my surgeon would be removing the tumor. If that were the case, I would need to stay in the hospital for five days afterward.

Although this was more information than we had earlier, it did not come close to providing clarity on what would happen the next morning. Even after being admitted into the ICU and hearing from a doctor, it seemed like nobody was confident about what the next stage of my life would involve.

For the next ten hours, I tried to relax and not think about my situation. We all tried to get some sleep, but none of us could. I was restless because my mind kept racing. I must have played out every possible situation that could happen the next day. Yet, none of them included leaving the hospital as if nothing had happened. The immediate danger remained a source of anxiety that entire night.

A nurse would periodically enter to monitor my vital signs, yet the room remained relatively quiet. Now, it was just a matter of time.

Let the Battle Begin

After a restless night, morning arrived. Around 7 a.m., a tall man with a gray beard and a computer on a cart appeared in my corner of the ICU. He approached my bed and said, "Hello, I am Dr. Honeycutt. I will be Christian's surgeon this morning."

Dr. Honeycutt opened up an image on the computer and began to explain what the emergency was. I indeed had a tumor in the center of my brain, and it was causing hydrocephalus. This condition involves a significant accumulation of fluid on the brain, posing serious risks. It can lead to seizures and other life-threatening symptoms. My surgeon mentioned that, in my case, there was an astonishing amount of fluid on my brain. I was a ticking time bomb.

I began to picture a *Drake and Josh* episode in which Josh accidentally made Drake's head explode during a dream. The only difference in the vision was that instead of Drake's head exploding, it was mine.

When I came back to reality, Dr. Honeycutt began to describe the procedure. He drew a line on the screen of his computer, illustrating the path he was going to take into my brain. He would go in from the top of my forehead and down into the center of my brain where the tumor was. His first goal was to relieve the fluid from my brain by poking a hole in some tissue. This would allow the fluid to drain. Assuming the first goal was successfully achieved, his next objective was to obtain a biopsy of the tumor, though there was no guarantee that this would be possible. Dr. Honeycutt explained that the surgery would last approximately an hour, and I would spend some time in the ICU following the procedure before being transferred to a different room.

After going through the surgery details, Dr. Honeycutt turned toward us, and I thought he was going to ask us if we had any questions. To our surprise, he asked, " May I pray over Christian before we start?"

My parents and I just looked at each other in awe. Immediately, God's presence blew through my doubt, and His presence was felt in the room. I was amazed and confused. It did not seem natural for a doctor to ask to pray for a family. I felt like something deeper was behind Dr. Honeycutt's actions.

We honored his request and bowed our heads as my surgeon placed his hand on my head and began to pray over the impending operation. A profound amount of peace filled the room and came over our hearts.

Dr. Honeycutt concluded the prayer with an "Amen!" He then told us that he planned to do the procedure at about 10:00, which was three hours away, and he would be in shortly before to answer any final questions we might have.

I now had three hours to mentally "prepare myself" for what was about to unfold, and the anxiety began to resurface. My head was about to be opened, and a pointy tool was about to be pushed through my brain. I had only known my surgeon for five minutes, and he was about to do an intrusive surgery on one of the most delicate parts of my body.

New questions came into existence. *What if this man, whom I had just met, made a mistake while guiding an instrument through my brain? What if he could not find a good place to poke the hole? What if he was unable to get a biopsy?* There was a possibility that things would not go right, and that was terrifying.

Before much more thinking could occur, my surgeon popped back in the room and said, "My next appointment got canceled, let's go ahead and begin."

Now, I had no more time to "prepare." It was game time! Nurses rolled my bed out of the ICU, along the halls, and into another room. I assumed we were close to an operating room. I was nervous, but I had no more time to dwell on the questions that augmented my doubt. My mind entered into a sort of fight or flight mode, and I had to place hope in the possibility that the God I had been doubting was in control.

Shortly after we entered the room, a man came in and introduced himself as our anesthesiologist. He then stated, "My priority today is to keep you safe and make sure your body reacts to the anesthesia well, the second is to keep you comfortable and make sure you sleep peacefully, and the third is this: I am a dad, I have three kids, and nobody messes with my kids. While you are with me, you become one of my kids today."

After he had spoken, I glanced at my parents, who had tears in their eyes. I can only imagine what was going through their minds. They were in an unusual state in which they had no control over their own child's well-being. And they were being forced to trust strangers to save their son from death.

For an anesthesiologist to make such a statement must have rocked their world. It appeared that the God I was struggling to put faith in was showing up for my parents, and He wasn't finished. The next words to come out of my anesthesiologist's mouth were, "May I pray over the surgery before we start?"

God Lays Fingerprints

Isaiah 41:10 (NLT) says, "Fear not for I am with you. Don't be discouraged, for I am your God..." God knows every situation we will encounter in life. This verse points to the fact that God is not a wall in our way but a support system to hold us up in tough times.

The experience of my worst fear coming true only deepened my doubt. Even though I couldn't bring myself to trust in Him, God showed my family and me that He was with us.

I think about my surgeon, who had probably done that surgery before. From the moment he began explaining the situation, it was clear he was confident in what he was doing. Even more astonishing, Dr. Honeycutt's desire to pray over us and trust God was sincere. We didn't have a theological conversation, but I could tell he truly intended to trust his skills and the outcome of the surgery to God.

My anesthesiologist's heartfelt words brought tears to my parents and me. My mom and dad could not be in the surgery to take care of me. I had relied on their care my whole life, and now they had no way to protect me. When my anesthesiologist proclaimed me as one of his own children, it showed us the love that he had for his patients. He didn't just view the surgery as another task of his job. Like my surgeon, he intended to treat his patient like family, and he rested on God's control in the surgery.

These interactions were just a few of God's fingerprints at the beginning of my trial, with the first occurring when we arrived at the hospital the evening before. Witnessing these acts of submission to God, on top of the trust that my parents professed, I was convinced that the only thing I could do was give the situation to Him. Although my doubts lingered, and I remained skeptical of His existence, a sense of faith began to take hold. I can only attribute this to God meeting me in my doubt and giving me the strength to trust Him when I needed it most. Over the next few months, God would place more prayers, encounters, and people in my path.

The Final Moments

Once my anesthesiologist completed his prayer, he began to describe the process of administering a relaxing agent that, for lack of a better term, would transport me to "Lala Land." They brought in a tube and injected the liquid it held into my IV.

We didn't have but about a minute until I would arrive at "Lala Land," so my parents began to share their final words with me. My mom grasped my hand and kissed my forehead, while my dad reassured me that I would do great. Whatever happened after that is a mystery to me. I had now entered "Lala Land." The battle had begun, and I was in the hands of my surgeon (in hindsight, I believe these were truly the hands of God).

CHAPTER THREE

*F*ive seconds later (or so it seemed), I was waking up to my dad and mom with smiles on their faces.

My dad said, "You did great, buddy! The surgery is over."

My mom and dad were both ecstatic. I had made it through surgery, and it went as smoothly as possible! My surgeon successfully poked a hole through the tissue near my tumor and obtained a biopsy during the process. I was very drowsy and nauseous, so it took a little while for me to comprehend that my life was, at the moment, no longer in jeopardy.

I spent the next couple of hours trying to figure out where up and down were and trying to overcome the overwhelming urge to throw up. It wasn't until the nurses gave me what I have come to call the "Big Kahuna" of nausea medicine that I reached a point of stability.

Once I could comprehend the world around me, I asked my

mom and dad what they were planning to do next.

My mom replied, "Well, they are going to send your biopsy to Johns Hopkins University in Boston, and they said we should know more about the tumor next week."

Then my dad said, "Yeah, we met your oncologist during your surgery. He is nice. You're in great hands, Buddy!"

Much of the events that unfolded in the following hours are a bit foggy. From the brief conversations my parents had with the doctors, we could tell that they were pleased with my oncology team. It seemed like I had reason to hope for healing.

As the fogginess from the anesthesia began to fade, anxiety and fear crept back into my mind. Eventually, I was brought back to the reality of my situation. While my life had been temporarily saved, it did not mean I was in the clear. My surgeon hadn't removed the tumor. He had just stopped it from killing me sooner.

Additionally, the prospect of having brain cancer was setting in. At this point, cancer was not a certainty but a possibility. Although the last thing I wanted was to have brain cancer, the uncertainty of it was a mountain in front of me. After approximately sixteen hours into my journey with a brain tumor, it became clear that the feeling of uncertainty would not be a one-time experience.

The reality was that if I did have brain cancer, it would cause more uncertainty regarding my chances of surviving this trial. Even if I did survive, there would be uncertainty about leading a normal life afterward. All of these uncertainties were intertwined as they revolved around the future. It became clear to me that I would face another foe in the coming months. As I lay in my hospital bed, I realized that I was dealing with the monster of the unknown.

The Monster of the Unknown

The unknown is one of the hardest things we encounter in life. It is challenging because it brings a complete loss of control into the life of its victim. While we can change how certain situations influence our lives, we inevitably encounter challenges and trials that are out of our control. In these instances, we can't escape what will ultimately happen, good or bad, and that is a daunting experience. When life is snowballing toward an unknown destination, it is hard not to become weary. Truthfully, the unknown gets its power by removing control from our lives.

I have deeply contemplated why loss of control is such a challenging hurdle to jump over. I think it stems from the fact that when we lack control over situations, the likelihood of encountering negative experiences, such as pain, rises. The reason why we want to avoid pain is obvious. We were not created to experience pain in life. The Bible says we were created to live a perfect eternity with God.

It was our misuse of free will that brought a curse upon our natural habitat. Since then, our world has been susceptible to things like disease, natural disasters, and death. These things are out of our control. They impact our health, corrupt our security, and end our lives. In my case, the trial had the potential to do all three things.

I read a verse the other day that said, "I am the Alpha and Omega, the beginning and the end" (Revelation 1:8). This verse highlights God's sovereignty over all things. He is Lord. He has the power and authority to control everything, and He will do as He wishes. Therefore, He has control over the very things that we don't. So, when anything happens, it is because God permits it. The Bible says, "God is love." The writer doesn't merely suggest God is the source of all love, which He certainly is. Rather, John maintains that God and love are the same thing!

When examining these characteristics, we encounter two seemingly contradictory concepts: God permits bad things to happen to us, but He is love. How could this be? I struggled with this question when I was experiencing doubt, and it would only continue to overwhelm me as I faced my trial in the months ahead. I hope to provide some clarity as this story progresses.

Here I was, only fifteen years old, met with the possibility that a full life could be taken from me. I remember that upon hearing the words "they have found a mass in your brain," I felt like all my plans and dreams vanished. I couldn't help but look death in the eye, and this seemed impossible at fifteen.

In terms of how the unknown presented itself in my situation, it appeared that there were two main outcomes:

A benign tumor.

A cancerous tumor.

In the instance of a benign tumor, the expectation would be an easier and more favorable removal process, leading to a shorter time of recovery. My life may change for a few months, but the side effects would be minimal.

However, if the unknown resulted in a cancer diagnosis, I would experience a much more challenging road to healing. I could be facing the end of my life, and surviving cancer would not leave me unscathed.

No matter what, life was going to look different now, and it would feel restricted in the immediate future. I was likely to experience pain, and my plans and goals were compromised. There was even a chance that I might not return to a normal life or experience a fulfilling life altogether.

Due to the doubt that had overtaken my belief system in the last six months, I was met with the challenge of putting faith in God. We had seen how those powerful prayers impacted different moments during my stay at the hospital. Despite this, I struggled to meet this challenge and fully trust Jesus.

When I looked at the future, there was no way to know what would happen. This was terrifying, and it caused me to feel like my life was slipping away before my own eyes. I only had a sliver of hope that if He was real, He would answer our prayer and save me from my tumor.

Deception of the Temporary

At one point, my aunt came to the ICU, so my parents could go eat a late lunch. I hoped that her jokes would cheer me up, but they didn't. Eventually, she noticed that I was feeling low.

"What's wrong, Christian," she asked.

"I am just worried. What if the results show brain cancer? I don't want my life to be over."

"Your life is not and will not be over. Christian, this is only temporary," she replied. "You may go through a lot in the impending future, but it is temporary. You trust God, right?"

I said yes with a sense of hesitation. Her words were wise, and I knew that whatever was about to happen would be temporary. But I still couldn't put my trust in God. He had just demonstrated His power through the prayers offered before surgery and the great work of my surgeon. Maybe I should have had more than enough reason to have faith in Him. Still, fear of the unknown was enough to deter me from letting go and putting my trust in God.

Despite feeling doubt and fear, I tried to focus on the words "It is only temporary," which came with my aunt's encouragement. The rest of the afternoon, I repeated that phrase to myself a hundred times.

At one point, my surgeon came to check on me and to update us on the plan for moving forward. He reminded us that the biopsy had been sent to Johns Hopkins and that we could expect the results within ten days. He offered reassurance with the news that my blood tests showed no cancer cells. This was good because if my tumor was malignant, it was a sign that it wasn't spreading.

I was glad to hear the news, but I was still apprehensive. The only thing that could have cheered me up would be news of a benign tumor.

For the rest of the afternoon, I distracted myself with my phone. I shared a post on Instagram detailing the events of the past 24 hours. As soon as I posted the photo, support rolled in. It was overwhelming. Countless numbers of people commented with words of encouragement. It was mind-blowing to receive so much support.

Another source of distraction came from the thought of possibly welcoming a new friend into my life. While I was lying in bed, my mom shared that a family friend's dog had given birth that morning. Our family friend texted my parents, offering to give us one of the puppies. They were Labradors, which happened to be my favorite breed. The dream of having a new puppy made the moments go by a little easier. I was just hoping for one more thing to ease the pain and fear I was experiencing. This gift arrived that evening.

My best friend, Jackson, appeared in my corner of the ICU. I was so glad to see him, but I was sorry that he had to see me in such a vulnerable state. His presence was nice and calm. He is someone who doesn't seem to worry much. I am sure it has happened, but I haven't seen it throughout our friendship.

Shortly after he arrived, a nurse came in to inform us that I would be moved to my own room. Before long, I was settled into a new bed, engaging in a light-hearted chat with Jackson and Mr. Andy. In that brief moment, my anxious thoughts and fears faded away. For the first time in 24 hours, I experienced a genuine sense of peace.

Eventually, my guests headed home, and it was time to go to sleep. I'd had a long day and was ready to call it a night.

The next morning, a physician's assistant informed us that my vitals were stable enough for my release. She mentioned that once the discharge papers were prepared, I was free to go home. However, I had to attend an eye doctor's appointment first. This was to ensure that the pressure put on my eyes by the hydrocephalus didn't cause damage to my optic nerve.

This appointment seemed important, yet all I wanted was to go home. I was tired of being at the hospital. I wanted to be back on my couch, snuggle with my dog, and turn the TV on. I was hoping the little evidence that supported my tumor being benign was, in fact, true. I believe that hope was what kept me calm.

A couple of hours later, we received the discharge papers, and we were on our way. The eye appointment was just a short distance from the hospital, and it was not long before we arrived. We walked into the waiting room and signed in. It felt like we had to wait an eternity for the appointment. I thought my vision was fine, and all I wanted was to go home.

We were finally called back and escorted to the exam room. Shortly after, a man entered and introduced himself as Dr. Packwood. He explained that the purpose of the appointment was to ensure that the pressure from the hydrocephalus had not damaged my eyes. He conducted multiple tests to assess their condition. Once he completed it, he told us that my eyes did not suffer damage from the pressure.

I was glad and started to get up out of my chair to run to the car, and then my doctor asked, "Would it be all right if I prayed over y'all before you go?"

Wow, did I feel dumb! I had been so impatient over the last

couple of hours, but it seemed like there was a purpose for this eye appointment. Just like the prayers offered by my brain surgeon and anesthesiologist, it seemed like something was behind Dr. Packwood asking to pray with us.

Embracing the Fingerprints

Amid anxiety, fear, and doubt, I believe this was another moment where God placed His hand on my situation. From the moment I headed to the emergency room until I left the appointment, numerous interactions occurred that I cannot simply attribute to coincidence. I believe many people were the vessels God worked through during my time in the hospital. We have seen many moments where comfort and peace appeared because I was in the presence of someone I loved.

The moments spent in prayer are significant. God knows the power of prayer. After all, He created it, for crying out loud! He uses it as a way to communicate with us, and He can use such communication for various purposes. As I have mentioned, the impact of these prayers was that they were powerful enough to conquer the anxiety and doubt that were flooding my mind.

Once again, my upbringing in the Christian faith told me that it was God. As I sat before the eye doctor, I truly wondered how the prayers of three different doctors could be a mere coincidence. As with the other moments, they seemed to point to God as well. Over the next few months, I would discover whether it was truly Him or not.

CHAPTER FOUR

*A*s I walked through the door of my house, I gasped in relief. It was not long before I was resting on my couch. I tried to cheer myself up by watching my favorite TV shows, but that didn't help. I was depressed.

There was a moment when my sister Lauren came over and hugged me. I don't remember letting go for the rest of that afternoon. She stayed by my side until it was time for her to go to bed. While I had always been aware of her love for me, that day made me truly understand how much I loved her. Even though I wasn't as comfortable as I could have been, her affection was exactly what I needed at the moment. Like any siblings, we fight, but our love for one another is unwavering. She was another shining light along my journey.

When I went to bed that night, an overwhelming fear of not surviving the night gripped me. Now that I knew I had a tumor, I was afraid of what it might do to me. Anguish and fear filled my mind. It was excruciating, bringing me to tears. My mom came to the rescue like any mother would and embraced me. She brought her phone and began playing worship music, and together, we prayed for the night to come. She asked me if I trusted God, and I wanted to. Thankfully, I made it through the night. It was nice to be home, but I knew there was a long week ahead.

Over the weekend, I rested as much as possible. Considering that I had undergone brain surgery the previous week, I believe I had a valid reason. College football kicked off that Saturday, and I knew I had at least one more week of enjoying it before learning more about my tumor. Watching sports served as a source of comfort that I would consistently rely on.

I attempted to distract myself from my circumstances. Although I was depressed and afraid of the possible biopsy results, I was in denial that anything was wrong internally. I tried to convince myself that this tumor issue would be just a temporary setback.

Despite my efforts to suppress those emotions, I wasn't successful. The fear of brain cancer that had tormented me since childhood weighed heavily on my mind. I hoped these fears were futile. I wished for these fears to be unfounded and hoped the biopsy results would reveal a benign tumor. Yet, there was an insurmountable wall in my mind that I couldn't climb or knock down.

On Monday and Tuesday of the next week, my doctors approved half days for me at school. Upon arriving that Monday, my mom and crisis counselor took me to meet the nurse.

Now that I had a brain tumor, it was important for me to become familiar with her. Although everything appeared normal, my vision was somewhat blurry, and I experienced a feeling akin to having my bell rung. After all, just a week prior, I had a sharp, pointy object probing around in my brain.

It felt somewhat uncomfortable when my classmates noticed my absence and inquired about where I had been. There's no casual way to inform someone that you have a brain tumor. Most reactions I received were expressions of confusion, often followed by a stunned, "Wait... what?"

I wasn't surprised by the reactions of those unaware of my whereabouts. I saw a few students who had learned about my situation and had reached out to me the previous week. I tried to express my gratitude for their supportive messages.

Most teachers showed empathy toward my situation, while others attempted to downplay it. In my classes, I had a considerable amount of work to catch up on, and I tried my best to stay engaged. However, my focus was on the impending biopsy results. With each passing day without a call from the doctor, my anxiety grew stronger. I constantly asked my mom if there had been any news, but the answer was always no.

On Thursday of that week, I had another MRI to assess the fluid levels in my brain and to ensure the absence of tumors on my spine. It was a tough one. This MRI took twice as long, and I found myself feeling scared about the procedure.

I had to update my playlist because the songs from my last MRI evoked unhappy memories and emotions. Before I even entered the machine, I was walloped by fear, and I could tell my mom was scared, too. But like all moms, she put on a brave face for both of us.

Spending two hours in a tube wasn't good for my mental state. It led my thoughts to spiral into a cycle of "what ifs" about my circumstances. I tried to find happy thoughts to redirect my focus, but I could only hear the "what ifs."

I find it challenging to express the depth of my faith during that moment. Comparing it to a rollercoaster captures its essence. Externally, I maintained my trust in God despite the difficulty. Internally, I struggled to maintain that trust while I grappled with significant doubts about His existence. I doubted whether He could or would heal me.

The MRI session finally concluded, and it was time to head home. I wanted to hop off the machine and run for my life. The MRI technician praised my performance and chatted with me about the Texas Rangers (I had worn a Rangers shirt during my first scan). Although I struggled to focus on our conversation, I appreciated her attempt to steer the conversation toward a more cheerful topic.

That night, as I lay in bed, anxiety kept me awake. I tossed and turned, replaying the day's events repeatedly in my mind. I attempted, for what felt like the thousandth time, to convince myself that the tumor was benign and to brace for a relieving call from my doctors the following day. Yet, nothing could truly prepare me for what was to come just 24 hours later.

The Results

The next day (Friday) marked ten days since the biopsy was sent to Johns Hopkins in Boston, and we had been told that the results would be ready within ten days. It felt like an eternity. I hadn't heard anything from my mom. During my last class at school, I received a text from her stating that she would come pick me up. This was unexpected as I thought she had to work that day, and my parents usually made me take the bus. Nonetheless, I assumed she was just being thoughtful, so I kept my focus on my studies.

As school ended, I walked out to the back and noticed my mom's van parked outside. I climbed in and asked, "Why did you pick me up?"

"Well, your dad and I got a call from your oncologist this morning and met with him today," she replied.

"Did they get the results?"

"Yes."

"Well, what are they?"

"Dad and I will tell y'all as soon as we get home," said Mom, "We wanted to speak to y'all at the same time."

My house is just a five-minute drive from my high school. Yet, the ride home felt like it lasted forever. My leg shook uncontrollably, and I was more nervous than I had ever been up to that moment in my journey. This is quite significant, given the level of anxiety I felt before my surgery.

We arrived home, and I changed clothes. When my parents shared the news, I wanted to be as comfortable as possible. Once everyone was settled, we gathered for a family meeting in the living room, likely one of the first of its kind in our household. Such meetings aren't common in the Englert family. My sister and I took our seats on the couch while my dad found a spot on the footrest of a chair. My mom sat in front of us on the floor, holding a piece of paper. The meeting was now in session.

My mom looked at my dad and said, "Do you want to start?"

My dad nodded and said, "Well, the tumor is malignant."

I nodded in understanding. I can't explain my emotions at that moment. It was a feeling unlike any I'd experienced before, and I hope never to have again. My mind immediately plunged into a familiar panic, reminiscent of the moment my mom revealed I had a tumor in that hallway. Whatever hope I had concerning the results had now been shattered. My fear of one day having brain cancer was now a reality.

I tried to understand why God would allow me to develop a cancerous tumor. I asked myself why He would permit a teenager in the prime of life to endure something that bad. The voices in my head started screaming phrases like "You're dying," "You won't make it to adulthood," and "Is God really there?" My leg shook uncontrollably, and the next words that came out of my mouth will forever be etched in my memory...

"Daddy, am I going to die?"

The Weight of One Question

Even though many years have passed since those words escaped my lips, my heart still sinks when I read the words, "Daddy, am I going to die?" I consider it the toughest question I have ever faced, and nothing could have prepared me for that moment.

I couldn't have imagined asking my dad if I was going to die, but I needed to know the severity of the mass in my brain. I wondered how much danger my life was in. Thus, I asked the question out of fear, hoping the answer was not an unequivocal yes.

I think my question went beyond merely inquiring about the chances of death. It affirmed for everyone the imminent danger that could threaten my life in the months ahead. This realization was overwhelming for everyone involved. At that moment, I realized I wasn't alone in this trial. My family was facing one, too. They were staring straight into the unknown, and they would have to watch someone they loved suffer in the coming months. I think that can be just as painful as suffering yourself. My family members were grappling with the possibility of losing their son and sibling, and they were guaranteed an emotional journey ahead.

The Weight of One Answer

Once my dad took a moment to catch his breath, he replied, "Well, your oncologist has given you a survival rate of around 60-70%."

A sigh of relief escaped my lips. My dad then turned to my mom for more clarification. She opened the piece of paper and indicated a number line presented by the oncologist.

"On a scale of 1 to 4, your tumor is between a 2 and a 3. Being the special boy you are, your tumor is also very rare. In fact, only 0.1% of brain cancer patients have been diagnosed with this particular tumor," she said, "It is called a Pineal Parenchymal Tumor of Intermediate Differentiation (PPTID)."

She continued, "Their plan is to treat it aggressively over the next nine months. This means we will have to pull you out of school, but they have a program in your district that will allow you to do your schoolwork from home. You will get a teacher who will come by twice a week to help with your work. There are a bunch of different paths they could take with treatment, and they will explain that more at your appointment on Monday. But basically, your tumor is so rare that they don't have any paperwork that shows how it reacts to certain treatments."

I felt a sense of confusion. My survival rate was promising, yet my oncologist didn't seem to know how to treat it. This made no sense to me.

"They are definitely going to give you chemo to start and then go from there," explained my mom.

"Will I lose my hair?"

"Yes, they said it is a guarantee that you will be bald."

Are you sure?"

"Yes, I'm sure."

Contemplating the Unimaginable

The conversation with my parents that Friday afternoon ranks among the top two of the most difficult I have ever experienced.

Throughout the week, I had been preoccupied with countless potential outcomes, yet nothing could have equipped me for the news I received. Being told that you have brain cancer is almost indescribable. And I can assure you that it led to many more challenges and fears.

Before receiving the news, I thought that knowing the type of tumor I had would alleviate the unknown. I believed the biopsy results were going to clarify how my doctors needed to treat the tumor and indicate what my future would look like. This belief was reinforced by my hope that the tumor could be benign. As we awaited the results, I held onto hope, uncertain if the God I was questioning would be capable or willing to heal me from a cancerous brain tumor.

However, learning about my malignant tumor showed that I was horribly wrong. The fear of the unknown only intensified. Sure, my doctors gave me a high survival rate, but it wasn't 100%. They weren't even sure how to treat the tumor. Despite not having extensive knowledge about my tumor or the treatment plan, I knew that the situation remained dire. My life was still in danger.

For all I knew, the treatment they proposed might be ineffective, and my time on earth could be limited. Coming to terms with this reality was incredibly challenging. I wasn't done on Earth. I was looking forward to all the things that life would bring in the future. I was almost old enough to start driving on my own. I was just a few years away from starting college. I dreamed of getting married and having kids. And now, there was a chance none of this would happen. I held onto the hope that the upcoming diagnosis appointment would provide some sort of hope for the months to come.

Room for Joy?

The only bright side was that earlier in the week, we were given tickets to the final Texas Rangers game of the season, accompanied by coupons I could use to purchase a jersey at the team store. With the game just days away, it felt like this would be my last event to look forward to for a while.

About an hour later, my mom let my sister and me know that Aunt Tabi, Uncle James, and my cousins were on their way. I was looking forward to this.

Shortly before their arrival, my grandmother (Oma) called to check on me. She is someone who cares greatly for me and is always concerned about my well-being. Despite my profound worry for my life, I answered that phone call with confidence. I told my grandmother that I was going to beat this cancer however I could.

During our phone conversation, she shared a phrase that would become one of the guiding mottos of my journey. She said, "Christian, you grab the bull by the horns and kick butt!"

For the first time in a while, I sincerely laughed. My grandmother is German, which is why I call her Oma. Her unexpected comment was the most random yet uplifting encouragement I could have received at that moment. The way she expressed it with her German accent added a special flair. She sounded both triumphant and confident. I truly wanted nothing more than to grab the bull by the horns and kick butt!

That night spent with my family was nice. We laughed and tried to distract ourselves from our circumstances. My aunt and uncle kept us all entertained. Once again, my aunt used her taser as a source of comedy. She pulled it out, crept up behind my dad and me as we sat on the couch, and activated it. Not only did we flinch, but my dad and I flew off the couch and landed on the floor. It's important to note that my aunt didn't bring the taser close enough to cause any harm. She just wanted the sound of it to startle us. It worked, and we laughed about it for quite some time.

God Moves Again

The next day, I returned to church for the first time in weeks. I didn't know what to expect or what people might know about my circumstances. I was nervous about how to answer any questions that might arise. I assumed that those who were aware of my cancer would attempt to offer encouragement, and I realized that responding positively to that would be quite challenging.

The exhilaration from the previous night had worn off. I found myself filled with questions about what the upcoming months might hold, and my doubts about God resurfaced, taking over my mind. If God was truly present, I wanted an answer from Him.

Upon our arrival, our church family greeted us as if we were celebrities. People hugged me, told me they were praying, and asked questions to help distract us from my situation. I was thankful for the love, which served as further confirmation that we would have warriors behind us.

We went into service as soon as worship started. I longed for a sign from God that He was there and in the situation. I tried my best to dig up confidence and worship Him; it was hard. And then my negativity was obliterated.

The worship team started the song Our God Is Greater by Chris Tomlin. As the first note was played, the room seemed to go into slow motion. The beaming lights from the stage seemed to shine as though they were from heaven; they were all I could see. During the first chorus, the words "our God is healer, awesome in power" were sung. I immediately looked over at my parents, who were in tears, and I started to choke up.

I believe that God provided the sign I had been seeking, and He did so in a glorious way. In the past, music had served as a source of distraction from pain. But that night, God revealed Himself through the song "Our God." I walked out of that service amazed and puzzled. I could not deny the sign I had just experienced. But I still could not reconcile why God would allow me to have cancer.

God's presence was undeniable. After experiencing those early moments where God used people to pray and be there for us, I returned to the belief that a personal, powerful being must exist. Yet, I struggled to reconcile how God could be loving while allowing me to be diagnosed with such a terrible disease. What reason could He possibly have for allowing my body to be tortured and damaged? Even if God chose to heal me, it was evident that I would still face the long-term effects of cancer.

Take Me Out to the Ballgame

The next day (Sunday) was the first time I experienced a rush of excitement in weeks. My favorite team, the Texas Rangers, was one win away from clinching a spot in the playoffs. Having tickets to see such an important game in person was a dream come true. The following day, I would be meeting with my oncology team to discuss my treatment plan, so I knew this would be the last bit of fun I could enjoy for some time, no matter what the future held.

This was not my first Rangers game, and from the moment we arrived at the ballpark, I soaked in the sights and scents that brought back some of my greatest childhood memories. The worries about my upcoming battle with cancer faded away, overshadowed by the excitement of the wonderful afternoon that lay before us.

Before heading to our seats, my family and I stopped by the team store, where I could choose a jersey to wear for the game. As we stepped inside, I headed for the jersey section. I already knew what jersey I wanted. My favorite player was Adrian Beltré, the Texas Rangers' third baseman. Not only was he regarded as one of the greatest third basemen in history, but he also played with immense joy and was loved by all his teammates.

I made my way to the jersey section and immediately noticed a red Adrian Beltré jersey highly displayed for everyone in the store to see. Among all the Rangers' uniforms, their red jerseys had always been my favorite, and I had long desired one for myself. I grabbed the red jersey from the rack and bought it. As I walked out of the team store, I was ready to cheer for the Rangers in their pursuit of a postseason opportunity.

As we were about to head to our seats, I was blessed with one more surprise. Before the game, we had been asked to meet someone outside of our section. Somehow, my story had reached important individuals in the Rangers organization, and they wanted to give me a memento to keep as I faced the unthinkable. I was given a piece of cloth that seemed to be wrapped around something. And as I opened it, I realized it was a baseball, signed by the very player whose jersey I just bought, Adrian Beltré.

I didn't know what to do with myself as I stood there with this gift. But we had a game to catch. My mom gently placed the ball in her purse, and we headed to our seats.

As the game unfolded, it was clear that both teams knew the stakes. Each player gave their all, resulting in an exciting, high-scoring contest.

One of the coolest experiences was witnessing one of the greatest power hitters in history, Albert Pujols, hit a home run. While I had seen numerous home runs by major league players, this particular ball soared more majestically than any other moonshot I had ever seen. The fact that Pujols played for the opposing team didn't even bother me.

As the final inning approached, the Rangers held a comfortable lead, needing just three outs to secure their playoff spot. My family and I joined all the fans, standing on our feet to cheer them on. After what seemed like an hour-long inning, we reached the final play where a ground ball sealed the final out, resulting in a Texas victory. The Rangers officially stamped their ticket to the MLB playoffs.

CHAPTER FIVE

I have experienced my share of challenging meetings in life, one of which was the discussion with my parents on the previous Friday. But that Monday would be the toughest meeting I had ever faced, as my oncology team would be discussing their plan for saving my life.

The night before our meeting was restless for many reasons. I had just experienced the high of getting a ball autographed by my favorite player and watching my favorite baseball team win their division. However, the anxiety I was feeling overshadowed my excitement, leaving me tossing and turning in bed.

I had no idea what my oncologist was like or what his thoughts on saving my life would be. Was he optimistic about winning the battle against the cancer in my brain? This question weighed heavily on my mind ever since my parents informed us of my diagnosis that Friday, and it lingered with me. I felt immense anxiety as we prepared for the appointment, fearing that his perspective on my tumor and treatment would be far less optimistic than what my parents had shared the previous Friday. It wasn't as if they had delivered particularly good news to begin with.

I also came to understand that the tumor and its treatment were far more intricate than my parents could articulate or grasp. Questions of every sort flooded my mind. If they managed to eliminate my cancer, what side effects might I face? Even if I survived, would I be able to finish high school and live a normal life? Would I go to college, get married, and have kids? I truly had no idea what to expect from the appointment with my oncology team that Monday, and I was fearful that the news might not be good.

That morning, when I woke up, I was still very nervous. My parents were probably nervous, too, but they maintained an air of confidence. My sister would not be able to accompany us on the excursion that day, as she had to go to school. Fortunately, the timing of my appointment gave us a chance to drop her off at school as a family before we headed to the hospital.

This may seem trivial, but I was very concerned about what I was going to wear. I was attending an important appointment, and I wanted to arrive in something comfortable, colorful, and new. Then it hit me! I could wear my Rangers jersey that I had purchased the day before. I must admit, I secretly hoped that wearing the jersey - especially since the Rangers made it to the playoffs while I had it on - would bring me some good luck for my appointment that day.

After we dropped my sister off at school, we headed straight to the hospital. The journey seemed long. I can't recall exactly what I did during it, but I know there was a lot on my mind.

We arrived at the hospital about 45 minutes later. Following our arrival, we engaged in a ritual that has become a part of every appointment I attend - we prayed. None of us knew what awaited us after this visit. While fears and doubts may have been echoing in our minds, we gathered our courage and turned to God for help.

We walked into the hospital and headed to the oncology/hematology floor. My mom informed the receptionist that we were there for an appointment. In response, she handed us a stack of forms to complete, along with a buzzer that would alert us when it was time for our appointment.

We sat among a group of chairs and couches. It had been less than two minutes, and I was already sweating through my Rangers jersey. I was nervous, and one of my legs was bouncing uncontrollably. My parents and I looked at each other, smiling, and my mom assured me everything was going to be all right.

After what felt like an eternity, the buzzer sounded, and a lady near a door motioned for us to go through it. My nerves went through the roof, and my heart was racing. It seemed that I was not hiding my nerves very well as the nurse checked my blood pressure and asked, "Are you feeling nervous?" My mom confirmed her question, and the nurse proceeded to take additional vital signs.

Once we finished, the nurse took us to a conference room, which seemed like an unusual place for a doctor's appointment. It wasn't long before another nurse walked in and introduced herself to me. Then, a man with dark hair dressed in a plaid shirt walked in, accompanied by a woman with dark hair. They took their seats, and he said, "Hello, Christian, I am Dr. Murray. I will be your oncologist." I shook his hand, introduced myself, and anxiously took my seat.

"It is nice to meet you," he began. "I want to start by telling you that I am a blunt person. I do not color-code anything that I tell my patients or their families." This declaration sparked some suspicion in my mind. If he was beginning with a statement about his bluntness and lack of sugarcoating, how alarming could the news that followed be?

He went on to say, "Christian, you have a very rare tumor called a Pineal Parenchymal Tumor with Intermediate Differentiation." Those were big words that I did not understand, and he could see the confusion on my face.

"This term is a scientific way to describe your tumor. What it means is that your tumor has both benign and cancerous cells in it. That is what makes it rare. It is so rare that there have only been five reported cases since 2000. This also means that the paperwork we have on the tumor is about an inch thick. In each of the different cases, the tumor was treated differently, and it ended with different outcomes."

My hope in the healing process began to fade. This appointment was not starting the way I had hoped. Just as I had thought when my parents first informed us about the tumor, I found myself questioning once more, "If they don't know how to treat it, then how will they make it go away?"

An Abundance of Information

My oncologist explained that they knew how both completely benign and malignant forms of my tumor developed and responded to treatment. But they didn't know how my type of tumor grew, so they were going to treat it aggressively in hopes of eliminating the cancer.

He then started to outline the potential stages that would unfold if the tumor responded as his team anticipated. I would start by going through two rounds of the most aggressive chemo they had to shrink the tumor. Then, they would have me undergo an MRI to determine if I needed more chemo or if it was small enough to remove. Assuming the chemo worked, I would then have brain surgery to remove the tumor. After the surgery, I would undergo full brain and spine radiation. To finish my treatment after radiation, I would complete eight more rounds of chemo.

From a broader perspective, this plan seemed overwhelming. I found it difficult to comprehend each treatment, but I placed my trust in my oncologist and signaled for him to proceed.

He then explained the possible side effects of the treatments, and those included:

- Chemotherapy- Nausea, fatigue, hair loss, a weakened immune system (this would mean I would have to stay at home to keep from picking up germs), and infertility.
- Brain Surgery- My oncologist didn't even attempt to venture into the vast amount of possible side effects, and he said that my surgeon would talk about those with my family when we got there (Yikes!)
- Full Brain and Spine Radiation- Hair loss, nausea, fatigue, processing issues, and the inability to produce growth hormones.

He finalized the details of my treatment plan and pointed out several potential long-term side effects. The first was a possible outcome of the damage to my brain, which could result in my missing out on college. If the treatment was successful, he remained confident that I would finish high school. However, he was concerned that the processing difficulties, coupled with the invasive brain surgery, would probably hinder my ability to manage the demands of a college schedule.

Upon completing the list of side effects, Dr. Murray returned to explaining the reason they were adopting such an aggressive treatment plan.

"Any cancer that returns in the same form tends to return more aggressively."

He then asserted, "With that said, if this tumor comes back, it will take your life."

The Weight of One Statement

No one can truly prepare for the moment when they learn that their life is in jeopardy, and I found myself experiencing a similar shock to when my parents first shared the diagnosis. My heart felt like it dropped six floors, and I couldn't help but choke up and sweat when I heard my oncologist say those words. I was in shock, and I wanted more than anything to be back at school and living a normal life with my friends.

But at that moment, it became clear that every plan I had for the future was fruitless. Regardless of what cancer treatment might entail, the mere thought of returning to school and playing the drums again was the least of my concerns.

We had gone from my life being in danger due to hydrocephalus to being saved by the ETV brain surgery, to facing the threat of a cancerous tumor, and finally, to the biopsy results suggesting I might never have the opportunity to live a full life at all.

One Last Side Effect

He then delved into a topic that had never even occurred to me. He informed us that chemo might make me infertile. Becoming a parent is a dream for many, and I was no exception. The thought of a day when I might not be able to provide my wife with children weighed heavily on me, presenting worries I wasn't ready to confront at just fifteen years old. I wanted the experience of raising kids and getting to watch them grow up. I had dreamt of having a family in the future, and I couldn't understand why I was already having to accept the possibility that it would not happen. I wanted to do whatever I could to ensure my wife would have kids.

Dr. Murray then explained that there was a method to preserve my sperm if that particular side effect occurred. He mentioned that one of the ladies present would provide the specifics.

He stepped out into the hall, granting a woman in the room the opportunity to take charge of the meeting. She introduced herself and mentioned that there were some matters to discuss regarding the process of storing my sperm. She then offered me the choice to have my parents step out while we talked. Uncertain about the upcoming discussion, I wanted to spare both my parents and myself from the discomfort of being together during this conversation, so I asked them to leave the room.

It was just the lady, whom I had known for roughly five minutes, and me. She began to explain that there was a bank that could store and preserve my sperm. This option would at least provide the chance of having a biological child if I were to become infertile. She then mentioned that I would need to visit a fertility clinic to provide my sperm. We talked about what that process would entail, and shortly after, my parents returned to the room.

After discussing infertility, we shifted to some uplifting news that truly put a smile on my face. My oncologist introduced us to my social worker, who shared that I was now eligible to receive a wish from Make-A-Wish®. She explained the workings of Make-A-Wish and encouraged me to start dreaming!

My mom and I exchanged excited glances. After enduring several hours filled with scary uncertainties, this news brought light into a previously dark place. I was filled with joy and started to consider what I could wish for. Amidst what seemed like the destruction of many dreams, an unexpected opportunity to dream emerged. This opportunity was made possible by Make-A-Wish.

After the appointment, my oncologist's team took us on a tour of their floor before we departed. I got to see where I would spend most of my time over the next months. As we walked through the treatment centers, I saw a lot of children being comforted by their parents. Some of the kids were too little to know what was going on, but most of them looked frail and sick. The expressions on the faces of the older children reflected a mix of helplessness and hope. I realized that soon, I would find myself in a similar position.

Reflection on Diagnosis

I found myself in a dark place, with my mind racing through every detail of the treatment plan I had just received. How did they know that the chemo was the right treatment? There was no way to predict whether the treatment plan would work, and I felt like my life was boiling down to the roll of a dice. Therefore, I didn't know if I could rely on doctors to save my life.

I realized that in the months ahead, I would need to summon some inner strength to endure these treatments. At that moment, I was uncertain about where that strength would originate. I had never faced anything like these treatments or this challenge before.

And the worst part was that the uncertainty of my situation increased once more. I came to understand that numerous possibilities could unfold, the majority of which were not favorable. Many of these negative outcomes could even lead to death.

It seemed that placing hope in God's ability and willingness to heal was the only option remaining. Based on the footprints in my first stay at the hospital and the experience my family had at church, I began to recognize the reality of a higher power.

In my life, I have witnessed people pray to God for healing without receiving it. This observation led me to believe that if God did exist, He was either unable or unwilling to heal. If we dismiss the first possibility, then it follows that a sovereign God must possess power over disease. This implication indicates that God has neglected those in need during their suffering, and that notion troubled me deeply. Additionally, what would motivate God to grant healing? What gave Jesus any reason to heal me? At that point in my journey, I was unaware that doubt is a natural part of faith, and I firmly believed that my skepticism would prevent the Lord from exercising His healing power.

If my doubt had no connection to healing, I couldn't find a reason for Him to withhold it. It seems logical that He would provide the doctors with the necessary information to treat the tumor effectively. However, my family and I learned that God's plans don't always match our desires.

Facing the reality of death is far from enjoyable. Since stepping off the MRI table, I had been forced to confront this harsh truth multiple times, and sadly, this would become a daily occurrence. My hopes and dreams were paused, and it became increasingly likely that I might miss out on cherished life experiences, such as getting married and starting a family.

At that moment, I couldn't understand how Bible verses like Jeremiah 29:11 ("For I know the plans I have for you," declares the Lord, "Plans to prosper you and not to harm you, plans to give you a hope and a future.") were true because of trials. And it would be a while before I would understand.

It became clear that many factors needed to align for my healing from cancer, and there was no way to foresee whether they would. The odds of cancer claiming my life appeared to be more likely than the chance of survival.

Preparing for Life to Look Different

Following a long morning filled with intimidating information, our appointment came to an end. My mom, dad, and I gathered our thoughts and headed home. That afternoon, my goal was simply to rest. I would start chemo in a couple of days, and I wanted to be ready for it. However, this plan proved difficult, as my mind was consumed with the reality of having cancer.

On the Tuesday before beginning my chemotherapy, several events occurred that would shape the journey I was just starting.

The initial event was a significant meeting that my mom needed to attend at my school. During my diagnosis appointment, it was determined that I would require some form of home schooling. Fortunately, I discovered that my school district provided a homebound program, enabling students with long-term illnesses or serious injuries to continue their education from home while remaining connected to their classes.

In that meeting, my mom arranged my homebound education and met the teacher who would visit our home each week. This provided them with an opportunity to connect and for my mom to share important information about me that my teacher needed to know.

My mom returned home from the meeting, eager to progress to the next phase of our journey. During the meeting, another "God nugget" was unearthed. She discovered that my teacher's only scheduling conflict was a weekly Bible study she attended each week.

My teacher was another important person in my life who could pray for my family and me. This is significant because these supportive individuals who prayed and provided guidance were consistently there during our journey, almost as if it were a strategic plan. I refer to it as strategic because it felt like each person appeared just before or after I encountered another challenge. My teacher was one of those pivotal figures, and I will share how God used her to minister to my family and me over the next few months.

Another significant event took place that Tuesday, igniting a challenge that I would have to overcome on my cancer journey. Our only task was to visit the fertility clinic to donate sperm. When morning arrived, I felt weird. In just a couple of hours, I would engage in something that I knew to be a sin. While striving to reconnect with my faith in God, I hoped He wouldn't condemn me as much as He would other sins in my life. After all, this was being done to ensure that I could someday have a child.

My dad and I reached the clinic lobby together. While he went to check in at the front desk, I settled into a comfy chair. A few minutes later, he approached me and said, "The lady said they have pornography on in the room."

This created an awkward situation. I had never looked at porn, and I was unprepared to respond to the offer of free access to it. Naturally, my dad and I agreed to tell them to turn the porn off. But I was a teenage boy going through a bummer of a time in life, and I was susceptible to temptation.

At that moment, I was reminded (I believe by Satan) of how I was treated by my peers in high school. They were living the wildlife, watching and doing everything their hearts desired, while I wasn't. I was reminded of how some of the teasing had spawned some curiosity about the things they watched, like porn.

As I reflected on these things, my mind spiraled down a mountain of bad thoughts. The temptation seemed stronger than me. I didn't need the "footage" to play in the room. However, I wanted it.

In the final seconds before I went back, I devised a plan to take my phone in with me and watch pornography without anyone knowing. So, that is what I did. I watched it like I was the only one in the room.

However, I believe that God watched me the whole time. He watched me try to hide from everyone, including Him, thinking that I was the only one who knew what I was doing. This could not have been farther from the truth, though. God knew exactly what happened.

This reminds me of Adam and Eve's first mistake. They had just sinned for the first time, altering the course of humanity, and they were trying to hide from God. Sometimes, when we hear that story, the natural response can be laughter. Personally, I find myself chuckling at the thought of Adam and Eve trying to hide. I can't help but think, "How stupid of Adam and Eve! You can't hide from God!"

But laughing at Adam and Eve is truly ironic because we also try to hide from God. All of us have sinned in what we think is "the dark," where no one knows. Yet, the reality is that God is right there watching us.

While I am now confident in God's grace, I also recognize that the choice I made at the fertility clinic carried consequences. This decision would ultimately affect my journey through cancer as well.

Final Moments of a Normal Life

My diagnosis appointment and the final preparations before I started chemo would set the stage for the battle ahead. However, there was one more significant event that served as a "battle cry" for us as the journey progressed.

Soon after my diagnosis appointment, my mom reached out to a friend who is a graphic designer. Together, they crafted a logo featuring a bass drum with the words "Rock On Christian." This phrase would become the battle cry for prayer warriors as we navigated our journey. Furthermore, my mom created a shirt for supporters to wear in solidarity with my battle against cancer. The front showcased the "Rock On Christian" logo, while the back featured the Scripture I referred to earlier (Isaiah 41:10), a verse that my family leaned on during the challenging months ahead.

CHAPTER SIX

*W*ednesday morning arrived, bringing an early start to my day. We needed to be at the hospital by 5:30 to prepare for the surgery to insert my chemo port and perform a spinal tap. This port would guide the chemo from the IV into my chest and through my body so that it could reach my tumor. After surgery, I would be moved to the recovery area and then to a room where I would spend the next five days while undergoing chemo.

My mom woke me up, and as soon as I opened my eyes, a wave of nerves washed over me. We packed my suitcase into the van and set off for the hospital.

I had a plan for the journey to immerse myself in some music and begin journaling about my experiences. Many had recommended this as a therapeutic outlet, so I decided it would be beneficial to heed their advice. With my journal and earbuds in hand, I was all set for the therapy. However, just as I was about to begin my music, a song played on the radio. As the familiar tune filled the air, I realized I had heard it countless times before. Yet, this time, the lyrics resonated with me in a way they never had before. One particular section stood out as especially significant. The words suggest that when the world is falling apart around you and the answers to your troubles seem far away, God is there to hold you.

As I previously noted, I had heard the song before. But it was at that moment that I truly identified with the message conveyed. The answers felt far away. I couldn't comprehend why a loving God would permit me to be diagnosed with cancer. Until that moment, I had never looked cancer or death in the eye. Up until that point, I had never faced cancer or death directly. In that moment, I felt as if I was holding on while God was telling me to let go and simply be held. Although I couldn't recognize it then, my life was not falling apart; instead, His plan for me was falling into place.

These lyrics provided me with a sense of peace, though sadly, it was only temporary. When I recall those moments of listening to that song in the car, I can't help but beat myself up. I feel that those words should have put everything into perspective. I often remind myself that I should have turned to those lyrics much more frequently during my battle with cancer. Unfortunately, I did not.

As you will notice, there will be many more moments like that morning when I felt engulfed by fear, worry, and pain. Instead of seeking comfort in the words of songs or scriptures, I attempted to cope with my emotions by denying my struggles or distracting myself with something on my phone in an attempt to medicate the pain.

Soon, we arrived at the hospital, and I was escorted to prepare for surgery. Just like during my biopsy, they would administer a liquid through my IV that would transport me to "Lala Land." As that moment approached, I prayed fervently for the treatment to come. The fear I had pushed aside when "Just Be Held" played was now resurfacing. I combated it as best as I could. Moments later, they informed me that the "Lala Land serum" had been administered into my IV.

The next thing I knew, I was in recovery from surgery. I awoke to the sound of two men with country accents discussing fishing, leaving me utterly confused. I didn't have the strength to open my eyes, making it difficult to identify them. Eventually, their conversation shifted from fishing to the tasks of nurses and patients. Since neither of them seemed to be addressing me, I assumed they were unaware of my consciousness, and I called out for my mom. They informed me they didn't know her whereabouts but reassured me that she would meet us in my hospital room.

After a while, they informed me we were about to head to my room. I opened my eyes and prepared for our journey. I was tired, and my back was sore. My bed started to roll forward, with the nurses pushing it as they resumed their conversation about fishing. We must have moved up a floor before reaching the hallway leading to my room. Upon entering, the nurses gently lifted me into the bed where I would spend the next few days. As we arrived, my mom and her best friend were there waiting for me.

My mom came to my bed and asked me how I was feeling, to which I replied, "Meh."

I was hungry, though, and I made that known. After considering my choices, I decided on a sandwich from Chick-fil-A. While my mom went downstairs to pick it up, her best friend kept me company, and we enjoyed some lighthearted conversation.

Shortly after, my mom returned, and I began to eat one of the last foods that would appeal to me for some time. I would soon learn that whatever I ate right before chemotherapy would make me feel nauseous afterward. It took nearly a year post-treatment before I could finally eat a Chick-fil-A sandwich again.

Later that afternoon, my nurse practitioner entered the room with news about the spinal tap. A spinal tap involves extracting fluid from the spine using a needle. This procedure is often performed during surgery and can lead to pain and nausea afterward. The aim was to determine whether any cancer cells remained in my spinal fluid. Fortunately, the results from the spinal tap came back clear. We took a moment to express our gratitude and praise God for the good news.

In the past seven days, there hadn't been much to praise God for; at least, that's how I perceived it. However, the truth is that my situation could have been far worse. I could have been facing a stage four tumor that progressed rapidly, but thankfully, I wasn't. Yet, my tumor was still malignant. In fact, it was not only malignant but also rare. The unknowns surrounding my overall condition remained, and there were no indications of it improving.

The beginning of my possible demise would occur at 6:00 that evening. At around 4:00, a nurse walked in and informed us that they were about to start an IV to hydrate me before the chemo began. I was nervous and still sore from my surgery. It was getting close to dinner time, but I was not hungry.

At close to 5:45, several nurses entered the room, wearing what resembled hazmat suits. They were pulling a trolley with a giant IV bag marked with crossbones. Watching them, I couldn't help but question what was about to be introduced into my body. If these nurses needed such protection from the liquid contained in that IV bag, how could it be safe for it to flow into my bloodstream?

Chemotherapy is essentially a form of poison. While it isn't lethal, its goal is to eradicate rapidly dividing living cells. This treatment can lead to side effects such as hair loss, nausea, fatigue, and weakened immune function. Nevertheless, the negative effects are often outweighed by the positive outcomes, resulting in reduced or completely eliminated cancer.

The Monster of Chemo

Throughout the night, nurses frequently entered to check my vital signs. It was difficult to get any rest, and I woke up the following morning feeling exhausted, nauseous, and lacking an appetite. Over the next few days, my fatigue and nausea only intensified. The time seemed to drag on painfully; minutes felt like hours, and I was utterly miserable. I attempted to distract myself by watching ESPN, but the segments were on repeat. Hearing about the same football game multiple times became tiresome. Moreover, I had no desire to eat; the thought of any food made me feel even more repulsed.

Although the details of those few days are somewhat unclear, I do recall several memorable events from my time in the hospital.

The initial event proved to be positive. Just one day after chemo commenced, my best friend's dad, Mr. Andy, came to the hospital bearing a surprise gift for me. It was an iPad! Although Mr. Andy wasn't the purchaser, the identity of the generous giver remains a mystery to this day. Nevertheless, it was a huge blessing!

While the gift was a material item, it represented the unwavering support my family and I experienced throughout my journey. This support was constant and significantly impacted every aspect of my trial. Additionally, the gift allowed me to watch Rangers games and attend church services. Since the hospital lacked the channel broadcasting the Rangers games, this enabled me to watch them online.

Regarding church, it would likely take some time before I could attend in person again. Fortunately, my church broadcasts its services online, allowing me to watch on Sunday mornings.

The second event I experienced was not as positive. During my first round of chemo, I got very sick. The fatigue, nausea, and headache peaked at their worst. None of the medications provided to alleviate the symptoms were effective. Even the most potent anti-nausea medication, often referred to as the "big dog," failed to help. I felt so bad that I wanted to cry.

At one point, I got up to head to the restroom. Upon entering and stepping through the door, I felt so bad that I immediately turned toward the tub and vomited. I hadn't felt the urge to vomit before entering, but my discomfort was so overwhelming that I thought, "Screw it," and directed myself to the tub to let everything go.

My mom rushed in after me, accompanied by a nurse. The nurse started considering the next steps to address my symptoms. Meanwhile, my mom began to clean me up. I recall sitting on the toilet as she gently wiped me down with a cloth. At one point, she said, "I am so sorry you are having to go through this, Bubba. I wish I could take your place."

Relentless Lament

I heard those words escape my mom's lips, and once more, my heart sank. When would these moments of hearing comments that left me in shock, speechless, defeated, and filled with regret finally come to an end?

Her words sparked a whirlwind of emotions and thoughts that flooded my mind. The first feeling I experienced was sympathy. Watching my mother endure the sight of me fighting for my life filled me with profound sorrow. In most situations, such as when a child gets hurt or deals with a minor illness, parents can often take measures to help their child recover. However, my parents were powerless to control the pain I was experiencing, forcing them to sit and watch as it consumed my well-being.

When I reflect on this, I can easily believe that my mom's words were genuine and that she sincerely wished to take my place. Over the years, I've spoken with many parents, some of whom are facing similar challenges with their children. Frequently, I hear a variation of what my mom expressed. It appears that witnessing your child in pain is one of the most difficult and overwhelming experiences for a parent, and I understand how my parents would have gone to great lengths to alleviate my situation. There were also several occasions when either my mom or dad expressed a desire to switch places with me.

I would never wish my trial on anyone. The idea of my parents having to endure my struggles was unbearable. Witnessing their pain as they watched me struggle was far more agonizing than my own struggle. Since the day I discovered I had a brain tumor, a persistent thought has lingered in my mind - that I was destined to fight this disease (though that didn't make the fight any easier). I had no clear understanding of why I was dealing with cancer, yet I felt certain that this disease had chased me down relentlessly.

The second emotion I felt was utter confusion. Throughout my life, I had been told that there was a loving God who created humanity in His image, and He wanted nothing more than a relationship with us. I had been told that He was the Father of believers in Christ. Given this perspective, if my earthly father experienced pain as he watched me face cancer, how could a loving Heavenly Father not feel the same way about His children's suffering? And what loving God, if He foreknew that His child would suffer and could prevent it, would stand by and watch?

My response to that question was fueled by the third emotion I experienced at that time: anger. In my view, the only logical answer was that God should use His power to prevent suffering from occurring. However, it was evident that He had chosen not to intervene. Even now, as I reflect on that moment, my feelings of disdain are unmistakable. I was angry at God.

These three emotions compelled me to pose a question I've asked before. Yet this time, I cried out from the depths of my soul: "Why, God?! Why?!"

Years have passed since that moment, yet I will always remember the precise instant when I posed that question. I couldn't foresee anything in the future that would justify the suffering I was enduring. I yearned for answers that I did not have...yet.

Although I knew somehow that I was meant to fight cancer, I was still mad at God. Did I wish He would just take my pain away? Absolutely. Would God reveal what that purpose was in the months to come? In ways you can't even imagine.

Persevering Till the Next Hardship

Until this recent incident, chemo was winning the battle. I likened my struggle to that of David facing Goliath, but unlike the ending in the Bible, I would lose. I was beaten, barely having any energy left - quite the dilemma since my body required energy to handle the chemo. The treatment also made me so sick that strong nausea would seem like an improvement. I struggled to force myself to eat and had little hope of enjoying food again. It seemed impossible to envision getting through the rest of the week.

The final event I remember from that week became a turning point. While I was in the restroom, I heard the unmistakable sound of my hospital room door opening, accompanied by hushed whispers. Uncertain of what was occurring in my room or who had come in, I hurried to finish up and opened the door to investigate.

In the middle of my room, alongside my uncle, my mom, and my sister, stood my cousin, Brittany.

I remember crying out, "Awwww!!!" And embracing her through a hug that felt like it lasted for an hour.

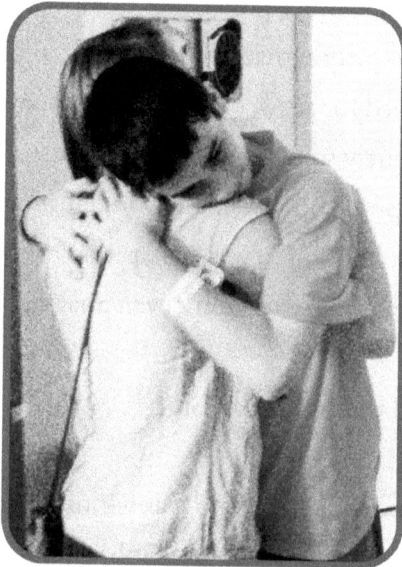

The fact that she was there completely astonished me. Brittany had just started her first year of college and chose to drop everything to drive 150 miles to visit me. That act alone reflects her deep love and support for me. Additionally, I know this visit wasn't easy for her. Until that day, she had only learned about my diagnosis through conversations with my family, so she was uncertain of what to expect. Nevertheless, she expressed that she "wanted to see [me], talk to [me], and give [me] a hug."

Before, I wasn't aware of how much I truly needed her. However, after seeing Brittany and hugging her, I came to understand the significance of her support. More than that, I recognized the depth of my love for her. This realization fueled my determination to persevere through the remainder of my time in the hospital.

The rest of the week proved to be physically demanding. However, thanks to the iPad and my cousin's visit, I felt mentally rejuvenated. During moments of nausea and exhaustion, I reflected on the support I had surrounding me. I fought through the discomfort, counting down the minutes until I completed the chemo and could finally go home.

With the weekend upon us, I had completed my chemo, yet I still felt weak. I was hopeful to return home on Saturday, but the doctor decided to keep me until Sunday morning to ensure I was healthy enough for discharge.

By the end of the week, I experienced a new side effect: my sense of smell intensified dramatically! I felt like I was pregnant, as certain odors made me feel nauseous (thank you, chemo)!

First thing on Sunday morning, the attending doctor came to check my vitals. After a brief examination, he concluded that I was fit to go home. Following a lengthy wait for the paperwork to be completed, we were finally set to leave.

I recall feeling so happy to leave. While we walked through the halls, the ability to smell every tiny detail didn't bother me as much.

I was free!

Traveling Through the Tunnel of Life

The day following my return from the hospital (Monday) was tough. By that time, I employed a familiar strategy as I aimed to relax.

Doing nothing allowed my mind to reflect on my situation. A wave of past challenges flooded my thoughts. While lying still provided me with a tolerable physical state, it left me lacking the energy to do anything beyond lying down. Over the past two weeks, I had been preparing for change, and now that change had arrived.

As chemo continued to make a new home in my body, it led to a decline in my white blood cell counts, compromising my immune system. This would make me more susceptible to viruses and require me to avoid public germs at all costs. Consequently, I found myself staying at home for the following month.

I was no longer preparing to be ripped out of a normal teen life. It had officially occurred. The activities I loved did not pause for me. My church youth group didn't stop meeting because I had cancer. They continued to meet on Wednesday nights, while I could only sit at home and wish to be with them. My friends were going to school and preparing for all the usual weekend hangouts, which included the high school football games every Friday.

Trying to cope with missing out on life conjured up the unknown. I had dreams of playing drums at my church on weekends, graduating from high school, attending college, and eventually getting married and having kids. There was no guarantee that I would ever do these things. The harsh truth was that I would be lucky to live. I was not ready to die. I truly had no idea if I would live to see my sixteenth birthday, and neither did my doctors. This tore me up in ways you can't imagine.

This situation seemed surreal. I had feared brain cancer my whole life, and I even felt like one day I would have it. Some might have called this an irrational fear, but the brain cancer had now occurred. I was now experiencing fear based on reality. I had no control over how chemo would impact my tumor or the outcomes of a potential brain surgery. This lack of control left me feeling weak.

Additionally, my faith in God was troubling me. Throughout the past six months, I found myself questioning His existence, and the onset of cancer only intensified that doubt. Nevertheless, I could still see the footprints of God throughout my journey. People arrived at just the right moments to pray for us, which demonstrated God's presence throughout this trial. I realized that these occurrences could not simply be attributed to coincidence. But somehow, those things weren't enough to take away my questions and anger toward God. I could not figure out why a loving God would let me go through a life-threatening disease. I continued to wonder if any good could come from my trial. My faith felt like it was at its wit's end. Unlike the kids we saw on the tour a week earlier, I was completely and utterly hopeless.

I felt this way inside, and at the same time, encouragement was coming from a direct source. During the day, my dad stayed with me because he worked from home. Throughout the day, he would check on me and do all he could to make me feel better. Almost every time he walked by, he would say, "You know that you are going to get through this, right?"

"Yeah, I guess so," I would respond.

I found it difficult to admit to him that I was afraid and struggling to maintain faith in God. In contrast, my dad was steadfast. This situation undoubtedly weighed heavily on him, yet he appeared to be resolute, placing all his trust in God's power and willingness to heal me. To this day, I admire him for his strength. He demonstrated confidence and resilience when I lacked both. He exemplified what faith looks like during challenging times. Although I didn't have the answers, I was fortunate to have the support necessary to fight.

The Light Appears

After spending the day reflecting on my grievances and professing false faith to my dad, I spent the evening looking for a way to distract myself. I experimented with various activities but struggled to find anything that would alleviate my anxiety and depressing thoughts. Then, the idea of reading the Bible came to mind. It might seem strange for someone angry and doubtful toward God to consider this. Looking back, I'm stumped by my desire to turn to Scripture. Yet, it seems there was another force at play.

I realized that I had fallen behind on a "Bible in a Year" plan I began the previous October. It's worth noting that my doubts about God began to surface when I committed to reading the entire Bible. As a result, I thought it would be beneficial to catch up on some of the chapters I had missed.

I went to my Bible app and opened the plan. According to the app, the next passage I was supposed to read was 1 Peter 1. I started to read the passage and came across two verses that said:

In all this you greatly rejoice, though now for a little while you may have had to suffer grief in all kinds of trials. These have come so that the proven genuineness of your faith—of greater worth than gold, which perishes even though refined by fire—may result in praise, glory and honor when Jesus Christ is revealed.

Upon reading those words, I was left speechless. The statements struck me like a semi-truck, and suddenly, a light bulb flickered to life in my mind. Although nothing physically changed at that moment, and I still felt sick from chemo, I could finally see the light at the end of the tunnel!

This passage conveyed three important insights about my trial. First, it served as a reminder that my experience was only temporary. Eventually, I would overcome brain cancer, which meant that the mental and physical pain I was enduring would come to an end. I understood that this could ultimately lead to losing my life, a reality I still needed to work through. However, at that moment, hope for the end of pain filled my heart.

Secondly, the verses emphasize that challenges are intended to strengthen faith. Over the past few weeks, I was certain that brain cancer would completely destroy my faith. However, the metaphor of gold being refined by fire suggested to me that God allowed my suffering for the purpose of strengthening my faith, not destroying it. Additionally, these verses communicated the truth that my faith is what God treasured through the existence of suffering. They brought me to the understanding that faith is much more precious than even the most valuable materials, such as gold, and it is the most important thing in our lives. This passage gave me the impression that genuine faith, which can withstand a storm, is the most valuable thing for God to sustain through a trial.

Thirdly, it suggested that trials like mine would result in praise, glorification, and honor on the day that Christ is revealed. By allowing my trial to occur, God intended not only for my faith to be proven genuine, but He would do something so great through my suffering that its outcome would glorify him. I realized that the greater purpose of my trial was to bring glory to something outside of myself. It was to bring glory to God. Did I know what that praise, honor, or glory would truly be for? Or when it would come? No. But I did know that it existed.

Beyond providing encouragement and peace, the passage in 1 Peter ignited the turning point in my experience with cancer. There was so much more fighting and struggling that would occur in the coming months, but this passage made it seem like there was growth and healing on the horizon.

CHAPTER SEVEN

*O*ver the next weeks, I continued to recover from chemo. My physical condition was deteriorating, and during a weekly appointment, we discovered I had lost a significant amount of weight. My doctors expressed their concerns and strongly encouraged me to eat anything I could. They even suggested adding butter to everything so I could gain weight. I had never heard a doctor prescribe a butter-filled diet, and I probably won't again. We also tried protein shakes. While they weren't my favorite, they provided essential nutrients.

Sometime after my initial chemo treatment, I started school with my first "class" in the homebound program. This turned out to be the biggest blessing! The program enabled me to continue my education from home and keep up with my grade level. The beautiful aspect was that I would not start new classes but would remain in the ones I had been in since the beginning of the school year. My teachers would send the assignments and lectures to me through email or my homebound teachers.

I recall feeling a little nervous on that first day, unsure of what to expect from my homebound teacher. I hoped she would be kind and understanding, someone who would support and advocate for me throughout the school year. With a lot of treatment and what I hoped would be healing in store, I was counting on her to help me navigate the stress that my schoolwork would bring.

Around 10 a.m., the doorbell rang. My dad and I hurried to answer, anticipating that it was my teacher. In the doorway stood a woman with blonde hair and a warm smile. She stepped inside and introduced herself, saying, "Hello, my name is Kathy Morris."

My teacher, dad, and I gathered around our kitchen table for a meeting. She started by sharing a bit about herself and expressed her enthusiasm for collaborating with me. Her demeanor was calm, relaxed, and full of joy. To wrap up our discussion, she explained how the homebound program operates and requested our schedules so we could choose the most suitable two times to meet each week.

From the moment we gathered around the table, my anxiety melted away, replaced by a sense of peace. Mrs. Morris' warm personality and optimism assured me that we would collaborate effectively. She had a joy and gentleness that lit up the room in a peaceful way. Although I had only known her for a short while, I felt completely at ease in her presence.

During our first session, I received some homework assignments. Thankfully, all my teachers promised to keep the busy work to a minimum. This meant a lot to me. Not having busy work to do each week would permit me to rest more from the treatment I was undergoing. By that time, it had probably been a week or two since my last dose of chemo. While the nausea had mostly subsided, I was still experiencing fatigue and a lack of appetite. My parents were exploring various options to provide me with calories without overwhelming me. So rest and recuperation were critical!

As I progressed, my sessions with Mrs. Morris were shortened to just two hours, making them manageable. I found it interesting that she had majored in and taught psychology. This proved beneficial because I faced mental challenges every day. While the physical toll of treatment was significant, it paled in comparison to constantly staring death in the eye, along with the accompanying stress, anxiety, and depression that came with it. In each session, Mrs. Morris took the time to gauge my physical and mental state before diving into our work for the day. Drawing from her expertise in psychology, she provided me with valuable strategies to tackle stress, anxiety, and depression.

Stress, for example, was an area in which Mrs. Morris had considerable knowledge and, therefore, could offer insight and suggestions. My doctors had warned me that stress could negatively impact the effectiveness of chemo in reducing tumors, which was concerning given the high levels of stress I had been facing. Eager to find ways to alleviate my stress, I decided to ask Mrs. Morris about it during her visit. Without hesitation, she recommended that I give coloring a try.

As a teenage boy in high school who was not an artist, my

hobbies did not include coloring. But I was willing to try anything to keep my stress level down. While I had reached a pivotal moment in my mental journey and was convinced that God was real, I still found it difficult to trust that He would heal me. This lack of trust caused me to rely on low stress to shrink the tumor rather than on Him. Nevertheless, I was interested in the idea of coloring.

Upon seeing my interest in this, Mrs. Morris brought a coloring book and a set of pencils to our next session. I was truly grateful! The calming effect of coloring helped reduce my stress, enabling me to work faster and more effectively. I even managed to finish most of my tasks without any issues.

Mrs. Morris was a knowledgeable and well-rounded individual. However, I struggled in geometry, and she didn't have a strong math background. After a few weeks of struggling with assignments, Mrs. Morris recognized the need for a dedicated math teacher. It wouldn't take her long to find a suitable teacher to step on board and get approved by the district. Soon, I would have my first session with Ms. Brenard.

In our first session, Mrs. Morris was present to introduce us and assist with any needs we might have. When I met Ms. Bernard, she appeared just as friendly as Mrs. Morris. However, I could sense that she was a bit anxious. This didn't concern me, as I was feeling nervous too. We were nervous together.

My teachers joined me at the kitchen table, and we began to get better acquainted. Before long, we dove right into math. I was three to four weeks behind and had to work hard to catch up.

Mrs. Brenard was an "old-school" math teacher. I don't mean to imply that she was old; rather, she preferred straightforward methods over the trendy, complex strategies that many contemporary math teachers had adopted. This was a blessing, as her old-school techniques were simple and made learning much easier. Facing fewer obstacles in geometry greatly helped to lessen my stress levels.

I looked forward to my sessions with Mrs. Morris and Ms. Brenard. There were moments when we wouldn't accomplish any work at all; instead, we would simply discuss what I was experiencing. Both teachers were strong believers and offered valuable advice on the challenges I faced. Their willingness to engage in conversation demonstrated their genuine care for me. Often, they were the ones who initiated these discussions. As I mentioned earlier, I truly believe that God orchestrated many relationships during my trials, and my connection with Mrs. Morris and Ms. Brenard is another shining example of that.

An Ongoing Wrestling Match

The time that passed since my first round of chemo brought noticeable improvements to my mental well-being. Before I got off the table after that first MRI, I felt as though my faith was dead. However, the mix of diminishing doubt and the realization that my greatest fear had materialized convinced me it wouldn't be revived.

From the moment we arrived at the hospital, God began to reveal Himself. Events like the prayers offered by my surgeon and anesthesiologist felt too significant to be mere coincidences. These moments served as a temporary source of encouragement to trust in God.

There came a pivotal moment when God spoke to me through a scripture from 1 Peter. This passage assured me of His existence and hinted at a possible purpose behind my trial. Although reading it did not resolve my problems, it ignited a deeper and more enduring sense of hope within me.

The uncertainty continued to prevent me from envisioning the future, instilling fear within my spirit. This fear made it difficult for me to find peace in the belief that God genuinely cared for me and would use my trial for the sort of purpose described in 1 Peter.

Throughout the course of my faith journey, a recurring theme has emerged in my story. I certainly experienced a fluctuating faith during my trials. As those significant moments of revelation occurred, I found myself in an ongoing "wrestling match" with God, a struggle that weighed heavily upon me. In the weeks following my discovery of 1 Peter 1:6-7, I felt compelled to confront the lingering doubt in my heart.

Fighting Doubt

One day, my mom came home from work and mentioned that a pastor from our church wanted to meet with me. I recognized him and have always considered him one of the wisest people I know. I expressed my enthusiasm for the conversation and asked her to set up a meeting.

About a week later, I attended my first session with Dr. Tracy Barnes. He is no stranger to trials and possesses an amazing testimony about his family. When you engage in conversation with Dr. Barnes, you may feel a bit less "intellectually equipped" than required. This isn't due to any unkindness or condescension on his part; it's simply because he is exceptionally intelligent.

I arrived at the church, and my mom guided me directly to Pastor Tracy's office. As I settled into the chair in front of his desk, I couldn't help but notice the impressive wall of books behind him (which didn't surprise me; all his wisdom had to come from somewhere). The presence of Pastor Tracy's extensive knowledge was crucial, as I was seeking answers to questions that seemed elusive. I hoped that his extensive reading and rich life experiences would provide the insights I was searching for.

He welcomed me with a warm greeting, and we started our conversation. He began by inquiring about my health and how I had been doing. Until that moment, I considered myself "healthy." Although I was dealing with a brain tumor and the side effects of chemotherapy, my vital signs and white blood cell counts were stable.

Regarding my current state, I shared with him all of what I have previously written. I had been struggling with my faith and the fact that I might not live much longer. I also expressed the disheartening reality that I may not be able to reach my goals.

Pastor Tracy's response surprised me. It came from a place of understanding. He viewed my anger toward God as a normal human response. He told me that it was common and that many before me, even leaders in the Bible, had times when they were angry at God. Additionally, he believed it is natural for us to be angry with God because we don't know His plans in their entirety. When we go through a trial, we can't see how it will turn out in the end. This is where faith is important, though. We may not know God's plans, but the Bible tells us that He has specific plans for all things, and they are good.

When it came to the possibility that my goals may not be accomplished, Pastor Tracy simply spoke the truth to me. None of us is promised a wife, kids, or a long life. We are not even promised another day. I remember Pastor Tracy using his own life as an example. He was in his sixties, and for all he knew, he would not live another minute.

This might not sound like happy, cheery news. However, we can rest in knowing that while we aren't promised another day on earth, if we have repented and are believers, we can trust in God's promise that we will have an eternity in Heaven where there is no pain, depression, fear, or anxiety. This eternity is much greater than the life we have on earth.

To finish the appointment, Pastor Tracy encouraged me to start meditating daily. Now, he wasn't talking about sitting cross-legged and saying "um" over and over. He was talking about meditating on scripture. This involves selecting a passage that relates to a challenge you're encountering and memorizing it. Once you've committed the scripture to memory, you can recite it to yourself when confronting your troubles head-on.

The purpose of doing this is not simply to memorize a verse. By committing a passage to memory and reciting it when its message is needed, you can train your mind to instinctively recall that truth in times of trouble.

In my situation, for example, I was struggling with anxiety. A scripture in the Bible that offers guidance on this matter is Philippians 4:6-7:

Do not be anxious about anything, but in every situation, by prayer and petition, with thanksgiving, present your requests to God. And the peace of God, which transcends all understanding, will guard your hearts and your minds in Christ Jesus.

I would start by memorizing the verse. Then, whenever anxiety struck, my plan would be to repeat it to myself continuously.

This was a great idea! While sitting in the chair and contemplating how meditation might influence my mindset, I became increasingly convinced of its potential benefits for my struggle with anxiety. In the following weeks, I started to memorize that passage from Philippians. Ultimately, this helped me find comfort in the belief that God can provide us with a peace that transcends all understanding, and He will protect our hearts.

Round Two

Shortly after I met with Pastor Tracy, it was time for another round of chemo. I remember dreading my second round because of how sick I got the first time. At one of my weekly appointments, my nurse practitioner told us that the second round would be easier than the first because I would not have a spinal tap, and they now knew what medicine to use against my symptoms. This was encouraging, but I still didn't know what the next few days in the hospital would bring.

On the day I was scheduled to check into the hospital for chemo, they ran out of rooms. This meant that I would have to wait until a room became available to begin my next treatment. In one way, I felt relieved as I now had extra time to mentally prepare for the sickness ahead. However, I also wanted to get this round completed quickly, making the wait inconvenient. At the same time, I was not eager to face the intense nausea, fatigue, and depression that would accompany the treatment again.

At about 8:30 that night, we received a call from Cook Children's Hospital informing us that a room had become available, and it was time to go! On the way, we stopped by Walmart to pick up some snacks. There have been several anecdotes about how music played a role in comforting me during my trial. Another musical moment happened as I waited in the parking lot of that Walmart.

While scrolling through social media, I noticed that an artist I listened to (Lacey Sturm) had just released a new single. Out of curiosity, I found the song and started listening to it. As the measures unfolded, I was captivated not just by the beat but the lyrics, which truly resonated with me. They were assertive and hopeful. They talked about how every day, we as Christ-followers are living the impossible. In my mind, this alluded to the fact that we were supposed to be dead in our sins, but because of the love and work of Christ, we are now able to live with hope in the eternal life that has been given to us through grace. This song encouraged me as I was going into my next battle. I thought about the bigger purpose I was fighting for. At that moment, I tried to put faith in God.

Once my dad and I arrived at the hospital, we went directly to the room where I would be staying for the next few days. It was smaller but felt a bit more comfortable than the room I had during my initial chemo treatment. My nurse completed the final touches on my bed, and I settled down, attempting to relax before they began administering the first bag. I also enjoyed some beef jerky, which, similar to the Chick-fil-A I had before the first round, I wouldn't be able to eat for quite some time after the treatment.

Shortly afterward, my nurse entered with the chemotherapy trolley and began preparing my IV bag. It was somewhat unsettling to see her dressed in a hazmat-style suit, just like the first time. By the time the IV was administered, I was exhausted, and soon drifted off to sleep.

The next morning, I woke up tired and a little nauseous. While I was much better than before, I still lacked the energy to do anything. At one point during the day, I recall my Uncle James visiting and spending time with my dad and me.

Throughout my life, I had known and loved my uncle, but we hadn't been particularly close. However, from the moment my tumor was discovered, he was right by my side. His visits to the hospital were frequent, and he did the best he could to lighten the mood. Over these months of fighting, his support meant so much to me. I gained an appreciation for the relationship we have, and I will always be thankful.

Because of the fatigue caused by the chemo, much of my time at the hospital was a blur. Other than my uncle's visit and a Fuzzy's taco I ate, the only thing I remember was a visit from one of my best friends growing up, Gavin. His dad, Chad, is my dad's best friend, and he is like an uncle to me.

I recalled my dad mentioning that Uncle Chad had shared with him that Gavin was upset because of my cancer diagnosis. From the moment they arrived, this weighed heavily on my heart. I did not want Gavin to hurt for me, but I was thankful that he cared so much. Throughout their visit, I tried to show him that I was strong and that I was going to be OK. We had fun and laughed. Gavin and I also caught up on life and everything that had happened since we last saw each other. It was a much-needed time of joy.

The five days flew by much faster during my second round, and before I realized it, Sunday had arrived. Although I still felt tired and nauseous, it wasn't as discouraging as my initial chemo experience. Later that morning, we received the green light from my doctor to head home.

A New Friend

Remember the puppy that the family had offered us on the day of my biopsy surgery? During all this time, she was in the back of our minds.

One weekend, just before my second round of chemo, my sister and I accompanied my dad to the family barn where the puppies and their mother were kept. At that time, my dad had no idea that the family had offered us a puppy. My sister and I planned this visit to help him develop a fondness for the puppy we had in mind so that when we shared the news of the offer, he would be more open to it.

We already had another lab mix named Gracie, who is a great dog. Every day when I would rest at home, she would lay by my side to make sure I was OK. But Gracie needed another friend, and so did I. This little puppy would also help brighten our lives as we faced the gloom of cancer. My dad was not on board, though. He is a dog lover, but in earlier months when we talked about getting a friend for Gracie, he said we were too busy to get and train a new dog.

While my sister and I were enjoying some quality time petting the puppies with our dad, the mother of the family walked into the barn to greet us. After a brief and pleasant chat, she turned to my dad and asked, "Do y'all know which one you want yet?" (Busted!)

My dad informed her that we weren't planning to buy a puppy. However, my sister and I quickly joined the conversation, letting him know that we had been offered one. Over the next few weeks, my mom, sister, and I dedicated a lot of effort to persuading my dad to accept the puppy being offered to our family. We even came up with a name for it.

Eventually, my dad reached a point where he would simply smile at the picture of the puppy we wanted. He even remarked that he didn't understand why he had been so adamant against getting the puppy when he was losing the battle. Gradually, he transformed from being stubborn to becoming open and excited. It wasn't long after my second round of chemo before my dad gave in, and we started to prepare ourselves for the bundle of joy that would soon enter our lives.

On a weekend in late November, my cousin Austin came to visit us. Austin is Brittany's brother, and he holds just as special a place in my heart as she does. Throughout my life, Austin has been one of my greatest role models. We've always connected over sports, especially Texas A&M football. I remember receiving a call from him while I was in the hospital recovering from my biopsy surgery. His visit that weekend was just one of many during my battle with cancer, as he would often drive from Tyler to spend time with me. This meant the world to our family, and I will always be grateful for the time we had together.

The Saturday of that November weekend, while Austin was still asleep, my dad entered the living room where I was resting. He mentioned that he was taking my mom out for breakfast. I nodded in agreement, pretending to believe him, but deep down, I sensed that they were actually heading out to get the puppy.

A few hours later, Austin woke up and joined me to watch college football. Shortly after, my grandparents called to see if they could come over for a visit. I happily agreed, and they made their way to our house. Just five minutes after they arrived, we heard the front door unlock. When I approached the entryway, I found my mom and dad standing there with our new black lab puppy, Aggie.

The moment I laid eyes on that dog, my heart melted. My sister, standing beside me, had a similar reaction. When my mom introduced me to Aggie, I couldn't help but hug her and love on her. I then took her to my grandparents and Austin so they could share in the joy as well. My heart overflowed with joy!

Aggie and my other dog, Gracie, immediately began to play. Gracie didn't seem sure about Aggie at first, but they soon grew to love each other. For the rest of the day, my family loved on her and did all we could to welcome Aggie into her new home.

I believe fully that God uses animals to bring us joy. I think He did that with Aggie for my family and me. We needed something to focus on other than my fight against cancer, and Aggie was that distraction. I also don't think it is a coincidence that she was born on the day of my biopsy surgery.

CHAPTER EIGHT

Over the next few weeks, I went about life much like I had in the previous months. I got plenty of rest, completed my schoolwork, spent time with Aggie, and attended my weekly appointments. Among those, two conversations held significant importance for me and my journey.

The First Appointment

The initial appointment began just like the previous ones. They drew some blood to evaluate my white cell counts, and then my nurse practitioner, Mandy, came in to check on me. As the MRI appointment approached, which would reveal the impact of the chemotherapy on my tumor, we had questions regarding the potential outcomes based on the results. We asked about the next steps following the MRI, and her response was, "Well, that isn't certain. If the tumor shrinks, we might do more chemo or just go to surgery from there. However, if the tumor blows up..."

Her words were interrupted by my cry of concern. The possibility of my tumor growing larger was something I did not want to consider.

The moment chemo entered my system, I did not feel good about it. Despite the newfound hope I had recently discovered, I couldn't shake the feeling that the treatment wouldn't shrink the tumor. This fear regarding the chemo's effectiveness led to significant stress and anxiety. When my nurse practitioner brought up the possibility of the tumor growing, it pushed me to my breaking point, and I found it impossible to remain calm any longer.

The moment I reacted, she stopped and hurried over to hug me. Then, she asked what was troubling me. I told her that I just didn't want to lose my life. "Christian, every day we have on this earth is a blessing from God," she replied. She went on to reassure me that since He grants us each day, I should find peace in His guidance and make the most of every day.

This brought to mind the encouraging words that Pastor Tracy recently shared with me. They emphasized that we cannot control how long we live or that there may be experiences we might miss out on. I understand that this concept may seem morbid. However, it is a truth that every human must confront. Acknowledging this reality compels us to face situations head-on instead of slipping into denial. When trials arise, we often struggle to accept the truth of our circumstances. The reality is that our days are numbered. No one lives forever. We cannot effectively fight a battle until we fully recognize the threat it presents.

I needed to accept the threat that I was facing, however challenging it was. While listening to my nurse practitioner, her words, "Every day God gives us is a blessing," began to resonate in my mind repeatedly. Since then, they have remained with me, profoundly influencing how I faced each day in my battle against cancer and shaping the way I approach every day now.

Alongside this, I began to understand the importance of relying on the promise of God's word instead of other "sources" of comfort. While some of these sources, such as my coloring books, offered a pleasant way to alleviate stress, they fell short of alleviating the anxiety and fear I faced. Other alternatives proved to be ineffective as well. For example, I found that seeking comfort in porn only intensified my anxiety. I fell into the trap that momentary pleasure could provide lasting comfort when, in reality, it only fed the anxiety that ultimately returned me to a state of fear.

Truthfully, God's peace was the only thing that could successfully medicate my fear, anxiety, and pain. There were days when I turned to Him successfully, but many times I found myself clinging to control and seeking out inadequate comforts. It became clear that I needed God's continued intervention to conquer my doubts about His plans for my situation and to trust in His guidance throughout my battle with cancer.

The Second Appointment

Another appointment that left a significant impression on me was with my oncologist. During our conversation, my dad inquired about the effects of chemo on my tumor. My oncologist explained that they hoped the treatment was shrinking the tumor and mentioned the possibility of it completely eradicating it. When my dad and I heard this, we both became attentive. He went on to elaborate...

He explained that while this outcome would be positive, it would also present a challenge. When chemotherapy dissolves a tumor, it typically leaves behind a shell of cells. In most cases, the cells within this shell are dead and are expelled through a person's urine; however, my tumor was different from the rest.

Due to the limited information available about my tumor and its surrounding factors, the doctors couldn't determine if the remaining cells were dead or alive and capable of multiplying. In this situation, my doctors faced the decision of whether to perform invasive brain surgery to remove the shell. If they chose correctly, this procedure could potentially protect my brain from a future cancer relapse. If they were wrong and the cells were dead, that would translate to high-risk surgery for no reason. Conversely, if they choose not to operate, they could be right in believing that the shell would be eliminated through my urine, or they might be mistaken, and the tumor could regrow.

Following my oncologist's explanation, my feelings shifted from believing that the chemo wasn't effective to also wishing it wouldn't be - at least not to its full extent of completely eradicating the tumor.

I didn't want my oncologist and surgical team to face the difficult decision he discussed with us. The uncertainty surrounding the situation weighed heavily on me. I wished for those who could influence my chances of survival to be free from additional unknowns. My hope was for a clear plan to emerge after my MRI results indicated the effectiveness of the chemotherapy, which ultimately meant that a tumor might still be present in all scenarios.

As I returned home from the appointment, I felt discouraged. Whether or not the tumor was still in my brain after chemo, I knew there was a long road of treatment and potential pain ahead.

The Impending Results

The next significant milestone in my journey was the upcoming MRI, which would reveal whether the chemo had reduced the size of the tumor. Until that moment, I had been occupied with school and taking some time to relax.

During that time, my fluctuating commitment to God persisted. I experienced overwhelming anxiety and fought it in every way I could. To manage my stress, I devoted a lot of time to coloring. In the week leading up to my MRI, my "classes" with Mrs. Morris and Ms. Brenard felt more like counseling sessions.

I sought guidance from God and reflected on the principles I gathered from 1 Peter 1:6-7. I also pondered the encouragement and strategies shared by Pastor Tracy. However, I had only just begun meditating on Philippians 4:6-7, so its truths hadn't fully settled within me yet. All I could do was place my trust in it and apply the insights I gained about trials from 1 Peter.

Some days, this approach helped me overcome mental challenges, allowing me to find strength in turning to God for comfort. However, there were also days when it fell short, and my anxiety would escalate alongside my feelings of doubt. On those tougher days, when I failed to seek God, I resorted to unfulfilling alternatives. I found myself trapped in this cycle, desperate for a sense of peace.

As I previously mentioned, I was uneasy about the chemo and sought clarity from the results. What if the chemo didn't affect the tumor at all? What would be the next steps? Would my experience simply turn into a frustrating cycle of trial and error with different treatments, ultimately ending with me dying?

On the afternoon of December 4, I had my MRI scheduled. I spent the earlier part of the day preparing myself by relaxing and watching TV with my family. Around 1:30, we got ready and made our way to the hospital.

One notable difference about this MRI compared to previous ones is that I would be in a machine capable of playing movies! Over the last few months, I developed an unhealthy aversion to MRIs. Naturally, they are loud and time-consuming. However, I believe the root of my fear stems from the trauma I experienced during my first MRI. Because of that experience, I could only associate MRIs with emergencies; they felt inseparable. While it might not eliminate all my anxiety, the opportunity to watch a movie during the MRI would help distract me from its results and divert my thoughts from the trauma I endured during my first MRI.

From the moment I woke up that day, meditating on Philippians 4:6-7 was essential. Regardless of the MRI results, I made an effort to express my gratitude to God for the day. I asked God to give me peace beyond my understanding. During the drive to the hospital, I followed my usual practice of listening to music and praying.

We arrived at the hospital and gathered as a family to pray before checking in. Similar to previous MRI appointments, my parents had a mountain of paperwork to complete. I settled onto a couch in the waiting area, attempting to meditate on Philippians 4:6-7. I had finally reached a point where I had memorized most of the verse, allowing me to concentrate on the truth it conveyed.

While I was quietly reciting the verse, a battle raged within my mind. I would focus on the idea of letting go of anxiety and seeking peace as the scripture instructed, but almost instantly, thoughts of potentially negative outcomes would creep in. Every time I would combat a bad thought with God's word, another negative thought would emerge. This cycle continued even after I entered the MRI. However, during the procedure, a different thought would arise to combat my anxious thoughts.

After waiting for approximately ten minutes, a technician came to escort my mom and me to the back to prepare for the MRI. I undressed and put on two hospital gowns, and then a nurse began to insert an IV into my arm. I chose to watch the movie "The Zookeeper." Since I had been using comedy to combat my anxiety, I figured that watching a funny movie, combined with scripture meditation, would be a powerful remedy. Before long, I found myself lying on the MRI table as the scan began. I kept fighting anxiety by focusing on Philippians 4:6-7.

During the MRI, I found my fear beginning to overpower the movie and the passage from Philippians. I was searching for ways to combat my anxiety when another verse came to mind - one my family had offered as encouragement since the trial began. It was Isaiah 41:10:

"So do not fear, for I am with you; do not be dismayed, for I am your God. I will strengthen you and help you; I will uphold you with my righteous right hand."

Specifically, the phrase "I am with you" kept replaying in my mind. Moreover, another saying began to resonate with me: "It will be OK."

The words I heard and felt didn't cure my anxiety, but they did provide some relief. My anxiety lessened just enough for me to endure the MRI. I believe that both statements were from God, as their essence reflected His character. They conveyed a sense of calm and resonated like a gentle whisper.

Eventually, the noises stopped, and the MRI technician entered to help me off the table. I was so relieved when the MRI was over. It was time to go home. I tried to push aside thoughts of the following Tuesday when we would receive the results, but there was no escaping the upcoming appointment.

We had three full days to prepare ourselves before the appointment. While waiting for the outcome of an event can feel like an eternity for some, that time seemed to pass quickly for me. Isn't it interesting how, when we anticipate something we'd rather avoid, time seems to fly by? Those three days felt like just three hours.

CHAPTER NINE

O n the morning of Tuesday, December 8, I woke up and prepared myself for the appointment ahead. I was uncertain about what the meeting with my oncologist would reveal, but it was finally time to uncover the unknown about the chemo. Despite my fears, I held onto hope that the results would provide some clarity. I hoped that my oncologist would have a clear plan for the next steps.

Just as I did the previous week, I listened to music and prayed during my drive to the hospital. I also meditated on Philippians 4:6-7, with the words "it will be ok" and "for I am with you" echoing in my mind. Once we had parked, we took a moment to pray before heading inside.

I recall sitting outside the oncology/hematology clinic while we checked in. Similar to my diagnosis appointment, it seemed to take forever. I was aware that many people across the metroplex were praying for this appointment. The anticipation of what we might discover felt incredibly burdensome. After roughly ten minutes, a nurse emerged and called us in.

We entered a small nook where my blood pressure, weight, and height were measured. After that, the nurse led us to the appointment room. I sat on the examination table, trembling uncontrollably. Every second seemed to stretch into a minute, and every minute felt like an hour. I mentally recited all the verses and divine phrases countless times. At last, there was a knock on the door, and my oncologist walked in.

The moment I laid eyes on him, I immediately observed his body language. He maintained a serious expression, yet it was clear he sensed that something was amiss. He didn't waste time with small talk. After greeting us and inquiring about our well-being, he took a seat and delivered the news. Echoing his straightforward approach from the diagnosis appointment, Dr. Murray stated, "Now y'all know that I don't beat around the bush."

When I heard those words, my thoughts spiraled to the worst possible outcome. I was certain my suspicions were validated and that the chemo had failed. Still, I held onto the hope that the next thing he would say wouldn't be, "Your tumor has gotten bigger."

"Your tumor has not changed one bit," he continued. "From what we see on the MRI, the tumor was not affected by the chemo. It is the same size."

I looked across the room to see my parents in shock. They were speechless.

Dr. Murray continued, "Our team has decided not to continue

with chemo. We are suggesting a resection surgery soon. In a moment, Dr. Honeycutt will be in to discuss the details of the surgery, but we suggest that we don't wait longer than about a month. We would need another biopsy to ensure that the chemo had affected the tumor, but the next course of action certainly needs to be surgery. We also understand that Christmas is in just a couple of weeks, so y'all will have to decide if you want to do the surgery before then. If so, Christian will definitely be in the hospital on Christmas."

My dad was the first to ask, "What are the chances that the tumor grows more over the next month?"

"Because of our limited information," Dr. Murray said, "we don't truly know the answer. However, in my professional opinion, if we do the surgery within three to four weeks, there should be no problems. I would not wait longer than that, though. And, of course, if you want a second opinion, we won't be hurt. Just know, I have been in contact with other oncologists across the country about the tumor, and they feel that surgery is the next step."

As he was nearing the end of his presentation, Dr. Murray informed us that my brain surgeon, Dr. Honeycutt, would arrive shortly. Before exiting, he mentioned that my social worker would come by to discuss the wish I would receive from Make-A-Wish and the possibility of experiencing it before my surgery.

Once he departed, I glanced at my parents, whose expressions remained unchanged. Their faces were filled with shock and disappointment, but I felt a bit different.

I shared in my parents' disappointment. It was disheartening to see my fears about the chemo results come to fruition, along with the belief that it wouldn't be effective. Receiving news from doctors that something hasn't worked can make it difficult to feel cheerful and optimistic. However, nestled within that disappointment, there remained a flicker of hope and optimism. As you may recall, my oncologist explained to my dad and me that a completely destroyed tumor would leave questions for my doctors. While the tumor hadn't shrunk at all, this outcome meant there were no uncertainties; they wouldn't have to speculate about the presence of additional cancer cells in my brain. They were confident in their findings and recognized the necessity for surgery.

A moment later, Dr. Honeycutt entered the room with an air of calm confidence. He greeted us warmly and took a seat to start his presentation.

"I am sure that Dr. Murray informed you about the surgery, and we are looking to do it soon. It will be a craniotomy, meaning we are going to take a part of your skull off to enter the brain. The incision will start at the top of your head, come down the back of your skull, and turn towards your ear. The shape of it will be similar to a horseshoe. We will invert the table so your brain will naturally split apart, which will allow us to go down the center of it. Upon entering, I will go in between the two halves of the brain to get to the center where the tumor is. What happens next is somewhat uncertain. We can't tell from the MRI if your tumor is attached to the brain stem, and we won't know until I get to the tumor. If it is not attached, we will suck it out with a tool and I will then have an MRI done."

"You can do an MRI during surgery," questioned my dad.

"Yes," Dr. Honeycutt replied, "We have a special MRI machine that we can roll out and place the surgery table in. I will use it to check the area and make sure I have gotten all of the tumor."

"What are the possible side effects of the surgery," asked my mom.

"There are several," he answered. "The first thing I have to do is move a vein that is lying over the tumor. If I strike it or move it wrong, Christian could have a stroke and possibly die."

This was starting "great." He hadn't even completed discussing the first side effect when death came into play. This statement didn't hit me as hard as the first words from my oncologist during my diagnosis appointment, though, and I was not too phased by it. I'm not quite sure why. Perhaps, at that moment, I was still focused on the reassurance that my team was confident about the next steps for my treatment.

"On the way to it, though," Dr. Honeycutt continued, "there are many areas of the brain we have to pass through and not damage before we get to the tumor. The first of which is the area that controls the eye. Even if I move through it correctly, Christian will still come out of surgery with a problem. It could be double vision, maybe not being able to move his eyes, or even an eye pointing to the right or left. We won't know which one of these will occur until after surgery. There are ways to fix these possible eye problems, which will be handled by Dr. Packwood (my eye doctor)."

After hearing about the potential side effects on the eye, I wasn't too concerned. From the way Dr. Honeycutt explained it, they seemed temporary or fixable. I figured I'd take my chances with some reversible side effects, especially if it meant avoiding a tumor that could be life-threatening.

"The next part of the brain that we will pass is the part that deals with motor skills and coordination," he said. "There is a chance that Christian's coordination could be damaged and that he could have trouble with fine motor skills."

Upon learning about the implications of this side effect, my thoughts instantly turned to drumming. What if coordination issues prevented me from playing well? Even more concerning, what if I found myself unable to play at all?

I jumped into the conversation and asked, "Will I ever drum again?"

"I think you will drum," he replied, "To what extent, I am not sure. You probably won't play at the same level you do now."

These words were difficult to accept. They served as a stark reminder that my hopes and dreams were threatened by the side effects of treatment. I felt I hadn't reached the level I desired as a drummer and was eager to enhance my skills. That year, I had dedicated myself to improving and playing for my youth group. This dedication had opened up more opportunities to play, and the idea of losing any progress felt like one of the worst outcomes of this surgery.

Dr. Honeycutt wrapped up his explanation of the surgery by saying, "Furthermore, as I mentioned, we are not sure if the tumor is penetrating the brain stem. If it is, the list of side effects I mentioned will greatly increase. My hope is that it's not, and we won't have to worry about them."

He ended his talk with a statement that really tested my optimism about the road ahead. After listing every possible side effect, he said, "You will not come out of surgery unscathed."

He went over the general details of the surgery: "We expect it to last ten to twelve hours, for you to be in ICU for at least two days afterward, and then a recovery period of about two weeks in the hospital." That timeline was overwhelming to think about. The previous surgeries had only lasted about an hour and a half each, so the idea of being sedated for half a day felt huge. And when I had chemo, just staying in the hospital for four days was tough. I couldn't even wrap my mind around what two weeks in a hospital bed would feel like.

I struggled to comprehend all the potential side effects that surgery could bring. While many appeared to be temporary or manageable, the idea of my surgeon operating in the depths of my brain was intimidating! What if he made a mistake? Had he ever taken that path to the center of a brain before? Did he truly know what he was doing? My life was at stake!

I had two questions that kept lingering in my mind, and I needed to ask them to find some peace regarding the surgery. Once he finished his discussion, he inquired if we had any additional questions. This was my chance.

"Have you ever done a surgery in that part of the brain before," I asked.

"Yes, multiple times."

This reassured me. I understood that since Dr. Honeycutt is a brain surgeon, he possesses a deep knowledge of the brain's structure. He would be familiar with the appearance of each brain region and how to navigate through them. However, even Dr. Honeycutt was facing unknowns in this surgery. The MRIs I underwent could only provide limited information about the tumor's position. He was contending with the possibility that the tumor might be invading the brain stem, which would add another layer of complexity to accessing the tumor. I needed to be assured that despite the unknowns facing Dr. Honeycutt, he remained confident in his ability to perform the surgery.

I continued my quest for confidence and decided to ask Dr. Honeycutt, "Are you confident in what you are going to do?"

His answer was a concise and confident, "Yes, I am."

That was all I needed to hear. Knowing that my surgeon was confident allowed me to have faith in him. While he also encountered uncertainties regarding the surgery, these did not diminish his assurance.

It's important to acknowledge that there was certainly anxiety and fear surrounding the upcoming surgery. It was a significant procedure, and numerous complications could arise. But I held on tightly to every bit of hope I could find.

Before departing, Dr. Honeycutt highlighted the potential dates for the surgery. One choice was to schedule it before Christmas, while the other was to have it afterward. He also mentioned that he would be on vacation prior to Christmas. Consequently, if we opted for the surgery before the holiday, he might not be available during my recovery. This factor would certainly influence our decision, as having him present would greatly benefit my healing process.

My social worker greeted us and recommended that we think about fulfilling my Make-A-Wish request before my surgery. At that moment, I felt "normal" and could truly appreciate what I wanted to experience. However, there were no assurances that I would feel the same way post-surgery. The potential side effects from the procedure might significantly affect my ability to enjoy the wish.

As we left, my parents quickly began discussing when to schedule the surgery. My mom wanted me to choose the date, and for her, it hinged on whether I was fine spending Christmas in the hospital. Conversely, my dad was a strong proponent of having the surgery before Christmas. Although Dr. Murray wasn't overly worried about the tumor's growth over the next month, his slight uncertainty was enough to influence my dad's decision. This was completely understandable; my dad didn't want to take any risks with the tumor. Nevertheless, both of my parents shared the same goal as I did: to have my tumor removed!

Preparation for the Unthinkable

From the moment we got home after the appointment with my oncologist and surgeon, we started prepping for surgery.

First and foremost, we needed to determine the timing of the surgery. Aside from the necessity of removing the tumor before it could grow, I didn't see many advantages in having the procedure before Christmas. There were two major drawbacks. First, it would mean spending Christmas in the hospital, which is the last place I wanted to be on my favorite holiday; I wanted to celebrate with my family. Additionally, there was another crucial factor that depended on scheduling the surgery after Christmas: I needed time to prepare! While it's true that no one can truly be ready for a life-saving surgery, I believed that having more time would allow for better preparation. I couldn't imagine how just a few days, or even a week, would help me find peace with the potential outcomes of the operation.

I was convinced that surgery needed to happen after Christmas. My mom and I managed to persuade my dad, and he concurred that scheduling the surgery for after the holiday was the best option. In a sense, it felt like we were taking a risk, or more accurately, a leap of faith, but it just felt like the right decision.

My diagnosis appointment and the final preparations before I began chemo set the stage for the battle ahead. Yet, there was one more pivotal event that emerged, acting as a "battle cry" that we embraced as the process unfolded.

Shortly after my diagnosis, my mom contacted one of her friends, who is a graphic designer. Together, they created a logo featuring a bass drum with the slogan "Rock On Christian." This phrase would become the battle cry for prayer warriors as we navigated our journey. Furthermore, my mom arranged for a shirt to be made for supporters of my battle against cancer. The front showcased the "Rock On Christian" logo, while the back displayed the Scripture I referenced earlier (Isaiah 41:10), which became a source of strength for my family in the months to come.

The truth was that my life depended on the surgery! While I had complete confidence in my surgeon and felt reassured that the next step in my treatment was clear, I struggled to find peace about the surgery itself. The upcoming month could very well signify the end of my life as I knew it. I needed time, mentally, to prepare for what I was about to endure.

In contemplating the risks and uncertainties linked to surgery, I realized there were specific actions I needed to undertake in advance. Therefore, I devised a "foolproof" plan outlining the tasks I aimed to complete.

First, I needed something positive or enjoyable to experience before my surgery. In the weeks ahead, I would feel an immense weight on my chest, so I wanted to engage in fun activities to distract myself and find some relaxation. I believed that being relaxed was crucial as I approached the surgery. I aimed to connect with as many friends and family members as I could before the procedure. The thought crossed my mind that I might not wake up afterward, making it important for me to say my potential goodbyes. Accepting this was challenging, but it was the reality I had to face.

Second, to truly trust in His protection and faithfulness, I knew I had to let go of certain things that were getting in the way. The first of those was porn. I realized I couldn't carry the heavy burden it created into the surgery. This time, unlike before, I needed to turn to God in moments of anxiety over the next month instead of turning to pornography for relief.

I also needed to release the lingering doubt that was hindering my ability to fully trust God regarding the outcome of my surgery. I believed that entering the surgery with doubts about God was not beneficial. Scripture supports this notion:

"Truly I tell you, if anyone says to this mountain, 'Go, throw yourself into the sea,' and does not doubt in their heart but believes that what they say will happen, it will be done for them. Therefore, I tell you, whatever you ask for in prayer, believe that you have received it, and it will be yours."

The mountain I wanted to move was the tumor inside my head. But I not only questioned His power to eliminate the tumor; I also questioned His very existence!

Third, I needed to discover how to place my complete faith and trust in God as I approached surgery. I began to feel that He was in control, and I realized I needed to surrender the uncertainties to Him.

Going Out with a Beat(s)

As the days went by, I started brainstorming how to achieve my first pre-surgery goal. Fortunately, we discovered that stopping chemo would enable my white blood cell counts to increase, allowing me to venture out in public once more. Thus, I considered various public activities that would bring me joy.

The thought of drumming at church instantly crossed my mind.

During the follow-up appointment, we learned that surgery could significantly impact my ability to drum or possibly end it entirely. I longed for one last chance to play before the surgery. So, I reached out to my church's youth staff to see if I could play the following week. They eagerly agreed, and I quickly grabbed my drumsticks, ready for one final opportunity to drum at church.

I remember attending rehearsal. Being in public again felt so unfamiliar, and I found it challenging to initiate conversations with people I hadn't seen in months. While I was certain they were aware of my sickness, I wasn't clear on what information they had received.

When I first sat down at the church's drum kit, a wave of joy washed over me, a feeling I hadn't felt in months, yet it felt completely familiar. It was as if I had seamlessly resumed from where I'd last left off. Each beat I played felt as natural as riding a bike.

The next evening was our youth service. I remember preparing for church and feeling concerned about what to wear. I had plenty of choices hanging in my closet, yet there was one aspect of my appearance that made me uneasy—my head. At that point, I was nearly completely bald, with just a small patch of hair at the back, leaving the rest of my scalp as smooth as a baby's bottom. This little patch of hair added a touch of humor, as its size and location resembled a yamaka. I couldn't help but think that if people saw me on stage, they might wonder why our church had a Jewish drummer, haha! Despite the chuckle, I still felt uncomfortable. Fortunately, many kind individuals had donated stylish beanies, and I found one that matched my outfit perfectly, allowing me to feel ready for the evening ahead.

When I got to church, I experienced another familiarity that had been lost in recent months. It was the worship team's "unite" time. During this brief moment, a pastor would share the purpose of the upcoming service, and we would engage in prayer together. I felt grateful to participate in that meaningful ritual once more.

After a rehearsal, we went right into the service, allowing me to enjoy another opportunity to play the drums with my youth group. The songs we played are still vivid in my memory, and I truly savored every moment I spent behind the drum kit. I played those drums as if it were my final performance, pouring my heart and soul into every beat on that stage. If this was indeed my last chance to play drums at church, I left knowing I had given my best and created a lasting memory I could cherish for a lifetime.

The Faithful Father

Have you ever heard the tale of the prodigal son? It's one of my favorite parables shared by Jesus. The story revolves around a selfish and rebellious son who insists on receiving his inheritance from his father, only to leave his home and family right away. He exchanged his family for a carefree lifestyle, which ultimately led him to a state of homelessness and despair.

In many ways, I felt like a prodigal son. Over the past few months, I had grappled with doubts regarding my heavenly Father's existence and struggled to trust His guidance during my trials. In response, I sought comfort and security in things that ultimately caused me more anxiety and despair. Although God had shown Himself to me in various ways, I still continued to wrestle with Him. I would run towards Him but then retreat whenever challenges arose.

The good news was that I began to find answers to my questions, and my uncertainty decreased. I thought about how God manifested in my family's life through the clarity provided and moments of meditation. A recent experience where I felt His presence was during the MRI. I mentioned the phrases that echoed in my mind, and I truly believe they were inspired by God. They carried a distinct quality, separate from ordinary thoughts, accompanied by an inexplicable sense of peace.

I was still facing a daunting brain surgery. It brought forth a feeling that had become all too familiar in recent months: a sense of uncertainty that led to insecurity.

Sure, my doctors were certain that surgery was the necessary next step; they had no doubts about it. However, there was no assurance that the surgery would actually save my life. In the days that followed our appointment, this uncertainty created an insecurity unlike any I had experienced before. I found myself yearning for clarity in the form of security. For me, that meant knowing that the surgery would be successful and that I would have many more years to live.

The problem? That is not how life works.

The prodigal son receives uplifting news: his journey isn't finished. Driven by desperation, he made his way home to seek forgiveness from his father, who had been waiting for his return. As the son approached the house, the father spotted him from afar. Without hesitation, he rushed to his son, welcoming him with open arms and accepting him back without the need for any pleas.

Similar to the prodigal son, my time of running and wrestling was now up. Only a few days after that appointment, I came to the end of my rope.

I experienced a day filled with nonstop anxiety. By the evening, I was drowning in fear and stress, desperately searching for something to help me feel better. I colored for a while and spent time with my family, but when it was time for bed, the thought hit me to seek comfort through humor on YouTube. This poor decision led to hearing a dirty joke that triggered me and drove me to access porn.

As I watched, I was overwhelmed by an immense sense of regret, feeling as though I had reached rock bottom. Lying in bed, enveloped in darkness, I was consumed by a whirlwind of shame and memories of wrestling with and running from God. I had never felt more mentally drained. From the depths of my soul, I cried out to God. Yet, unlike during my chemo, a different response unfolded this time.

Amid dark isolation, I looked up and realized I was not alone. Before me stood a Man with His hand extended toward me. While this may seem like a dream or a vision, such descriptions fall short of capturing the reality of the experience. The Man did not reveal His name, nor could I describe His physical attributes, yet deep within my heart, I recognized that I was staring directly into the eyes of God.

It was clear that I needed to take the hand of my eternal, divine Father, and that's exactly what I did. Although I don't recall any physical movement, I sincerely and wholeheartedly embraced Him in my mind and spirit. Instantly, a profound sense of peace enveloped me. This peace was different from what I had felt during my appointment a few days prior; it was a deep security that surpassed any worries I had faced in the last twelve hours.

I credit this moment to the time when I truly returned to God. Like a prodigal son who finally stopped running, I had been in a lengthy period of wrestling with Him, but I was eventually brought to a standstill. In His grace, God revealed Himself and called me to stop running. He showed me that I would not know the surgery's outcome before it took place, and I needed to place my trust in Him. So, that's exactly what I did. With heartfelt sincerity, I entrusted my faith to Him and surrendered to whatever the result of the surgery might be.

Genuine Faith Forward

Over the next few weeks, I somehow managed to stay away from porn. In moments of anxiety, I focused on the verses from Philippians 4 and did my best to turn to God. I truly believe it was His strength that helped me resist temptation. It was clear He had His hand on my heart, and I found peace in the protection He provided. Still, I knew there was something more I wanted to do, something I could accomplish: to move forward with genuine faith in God.

Let's revisit the scripture that resonated with me following my first chemo treatment. As you may recall, it was 1 Peter 1:6-7 that illuminated my thoughts and sparked a realization. This passage instilled hope within me, affirming that my trial had significance. Additionally, it emphasized the value of sincere faith.

I believe it's essential to emphasize that God does not demand a specific quantity of faith from us. Our faith isn't something that can be measured like liquid in a cup, with a line indicating the minimum required for it to be valid. As Jesus stated, "If you have faith as small as a mustard seed, you can say to this mulberry tree, 'Be uprooted and planted in the sea,' and it will obey you." If just a small amount of faith is sufficient for God to accomplish remarkable things, then what truly defines faith as good or genuine?

I believe that the quality of genuineness is what renders faith authentic. The passage in 1 Peter highlights that one purpose of trials is to demonstrate the authenticity of faith. Furthermore, James 1:5-7 cautions those seeking God's provision to approach their requests with unwavering belief rather than doubt. Doubt undermines faith, resulting in instability and a divided mind.

Let me clarify something important. The presence of doubt itself is not inherently wrong or sinful. As humans, we are not omniscient. I believe that our capacity for doubt can sometimes act as a signal that something may not be true or worthy of our pursuit. The real issue arises when we fail to examine our doubts, allow them to hinder our faith, and let them drive us to distance ourselves from God. That's exactly what I experienced during the six months leading up to my decision to return to Him.

I don't want to give the impression that true faith will always grant us our desires or alleviate our struggles. Acknowledging this can be challenging. My parents prayed fervently for chemotherapy to reduce my tumor, yet that was not in God's plan. So, why is it still valuable to trust in God when He doesn't always heal us as we wish, or at all? I believe it's because authentic faith and surrender allow our hearts to be open to God's intention to guide us through whatever He permits.

You might still wonder why God allows trials and tragedy to happen. The reality is that pain still exists, even when He's carrying us through it. But thankfully, there's another layer to this truth that I hope to shed light on by the end of this book.

During those weeks, I realized I needed to let go of all control and place my trust in God for the surgery and its outcome. I hope you'll see how that trust was truly realized, and I believe the strength to do so came from Him. As we continue with the story, I hope you'll recognize how God carried us through the immense challenge of the surgery.

The Support of Warriors

From the moment I stepped off the table after that first MRI, a powerful army of warriors surrounded us in prayer. Of course, there was our extended family that made up a whole regiment, lifting us before God's throne every single day. I think of my grandparents, aunts, uncles, and cousins, who prayed without pause. Some of them lived in Houston, others in the remote corners of East Texas, but it didn't matter where they were. Then there was our church family, who stayed in constant contact with us, and even people we'd never met following our journey on CaringBridge. Whenever an update went out, they all prayed earnestly.

I call these groups "regiments" in an army because their prayers were powerful, and they spread the call for prayer across the country—literally. In other states, people were praying for my situation. Strangers were fighting for me, wielding one of the most powerful weapons God can give: prayer!

I'm convinced that prayer is more than just talking to God, though that's certainly important. Prayer gives God's people, whether individually or together, a way to cry out to Him for help in the situations they face. When people come together to pray for a specific purpose, it's incredibly effective. As the book of James says, "The prayer of a righteous person is powerful and effective."

People were gathering together in Jesus' name to ask God to heal me, and the ways He had shown up were evidence that He was with us.

One of the most meaningful moments of prayer came when a friend from church came to our home specifically to pray for the upcoming surgery. Before she arrived, my mom mentioned that she had a special gift. She said Catie could move a room with her prayers like no one else she had ever met. That got me curious to meet Catie and pray with her, but I had no idea just how powerful that experience would be.

When Catie arrived, I was surprised. She seemed to be about five feet tall and as sweet as could be. At first glance, she didn't exactly fit the image of a throne-pounding prayer warrior for God. But I would soon discover that her appearance was no match for the spiritual fire that came pouring out of her soul.

We sat in a circle, and Catie began to speak words of deep wisdom. She shared her own story about needing open-heart surgery, but the challenge was that she had an important trip to take, one she felt couldn't be missed. So, she prayed for God to heal her heart in a way that doctors couldn't explain. Sure enough, at her pre-surgery appointment, the doctor found that the issue with her heart had completely disappeared. It was a miracle he couldn't explain, and just like that, she went on her trip.

Her story was incredibly inspiring. As she shared it, I could see the strength of her faith in God radiating through her. Even before we began praying, I could sense that she had a unique gift for leading others in prayer. She asked us to take each other's hands and explained that we'd go around the circle, each person praying in turn, and then she would close it out. As we joined hands, I had no idea what was about to unfold, but what happened next was truly amazing.

The moment our hands touched, and I closed my eyes, a wave of emotions washed over me. I felt an overwhelming sense of peace, but there was also a feeling of unrest, though it wasn't negative. It was more like something deep inside me was stirring, shifting. One by one, my family began to pray, each person laying out their thoughts, struggles, gratitude, and hopes before God. Their prayers were raw, real, and completely genuine. It was clear that their hearts were fully open.

Before long, it was my turn to pray. A need for God and hope were the basis of my prayer. I also thanked Him for the ways He had already shown up.

As I prayed, the story of the Israelites crossing the Red Sea came to mind. I remembered how God parted that giant body of water, making a way where there was no way. If He could do that, and I had faith that He did, then what was my tumor in comparison? If He had the power to control nature itself, how could He not be powerful enough to remove a swelling of cells in a fifteen-year-old's brain? I referenced that miracle in my prayer. I told God that I had faith in His power to guide my surgeon to remove the tumor that was a threat to me but not to Him.

When I finished, Catie began to close out the prayer. It felt like she spent minutes just pouring out every praise she could think of for God. She praised Him for the healing He had done in the past and for the healing she had faith He would bring in the future. She also praised God for His presence, which was already so evident in that room. She prayed for peace over my family as we faced the coming weeks and the surgery ahead. The words that came from her felt like fire—passionate and powerful. I truly believe the Holy Spirit was speaking through Catie during that prayer.

A Bonus Beat and Interaction

As surgery approached, I did everything I could to prepare myself for what was coming. But then, one day, I was given an opportunity that left me completely speechless. I was at home when the phone rang. It was one of the worship leaders from my church. He started by asking how I was feeling, and then he went straight to the reason he was calling. He told me that the worship team was planning for the Christmas services that year, and they had decided to ask me to be the percussionist. He then asked if I'd be willing to play. Without hesitation, I enthusiastically accepted!

I was ecstatic! This was, without a doubt, the biggest playing opportunity I'd ever had. It was a dream come true. It meant so much to me to have the chance to play in such a big setting one last time. Being able to play with the band almost made me feel like a normal kid again. When I was behind the drum kit or on the percussion stand, I wasn't thinking about the cancer that had kept me homebound for so long. Instead, I was having fun and doing one of the things I loved most.

Something I'll remember the most about playing percussion at the Christmas services was what happened after the last service. It was a moment that reflected just how incredible the support from my family and church really was.

As we started the walkout music in the final service, I noticed my lead pastor's wife run backstage after him. We kept playing, and I went on with the music, but I couldn't help but notice that they suddenly appeared on the side of the stage. As soon as we hit the last note, they walked over to my riser and greeted me. My pastor asked how I was doing, then opened his arms for a hug. He told me that he and his wife were praying for my family and me daily, and he encouraged me to keep fighting. The fact that they took the time to check on me right after the service was a powerful reminder of the unwavering support my family and I had.

This wasn't the first time my pastor showed that his family truly cared about what mine was going through. Over the past few months, my mom mentioned that he would often walk into her office just to check on us. What made this especially significant was that my pastor is an incredibly busy man. He's a best-selling author, travels across the country to speak, and pastors a church with over 20,000 members. For him to carve out time from his packed schedule to check on us in such a personal way was incredibly thoughtful. And that encounter at the Christmas service was just another reminder of the constant support we had from him and his family.

The Final Days

After a long and life-changing month, we were down to just a week and a half before surgery. The event that kicked off those final days was Christmas. It was a bittersweet time. My family has always been big on tradition, and we take the holiday seriously. Christmas has always been one of the most important times of the year for us, and for obvious reasons, this one felt different. We knew it could be the last time we'd all be together for Christmas as a full family. Even if I survived the surgery, there was no guarantee I would have the cognitive or emotional ability to fully enjoy future holidays. The weight of it all was heavy, and it was felt deeply by everyone in my family.

I remember a fifteen-second conversation that perfectly captured the weight of the situation. Growing up, our family didn't have a lot of money, and there were some tough times. But my parents have always been intentional gift-givers. No matter what our finances looked like each year, they made sure to put a huge emphasis on giving my sister and me a meaningful Christmas.

One day, my mom walked through the living room and asked, "Is there anything I can do to make this a nice Christmas for you? Are there any other gifts that would put a smile on your face?"

In an attempt to be cute, I responded, "My tumor gone."

This caused my mom to get choked up. In a sort of chuckle/cry, she responded, "I want that too, Bubba! I want that too!"

By now, I hope I've shown how deeply this trial affected my family. Through every tough appointment and difficult moment, my parents held up a strong front. I honestly don't know how they did it, but I do know they were facing something no parent should ever have to face. And while we can now look back and reminisce about those fifteen seconds, I understand that they reflected my mom's deepest wish for her son: that I would no longer suffer and would have the chance to live a full, healthy life.

As Christmas came and went, we embraced every moment we had together. Oma came to stay with us, and we shared countless moments with our extended family. We found comfort in each other's arms, and honestly, it was one of the most beautiful Christmases I've ever experienced. I don't think my family and I had ever bonded during a holiday in quite the same way as we did that year.

Pre-Op Appointment

Just a few days before surgery, my mom and I went to the hospital for my pre-op appointment. During the visit, one of the operating room nurses took all my vitals and walked us through the logistics for surgery day. The reality of having a life-altering surgery had already begun to sink in, but for the first time, it truly felt real. The final preparations were being made, and it suddenly hit me. At the appointment, we learned everything there was to know about the surgery—except, of course, how to perform it ourselves.

I remember how she walked in and said, "Well, I see on my chart that we are going to remove this little bugger, right?"

My mom and I just looked at each other and smiled because of the unexpected words from the nurse. The room went from completely serious to serious with a touch of light-heartedness.

The nurse then walked us through the logistics. Surgery day would begin for us at 5:30 in the morning. This was not when we needed to wake up but when we needed to arrive at the hospital. Once we got there, we'd check in at surgery prep and be led to a room. From there, they would check every vital sign imaginable and start the first of three IVs. After that, my surgeon would come in for a final check-up, go over the surgery plan one last time, and then it would be time for the procedure. Once surgery was completed, I'd be moved to the ICU for initial recovery.

Along with the logistics, the nurse went over a few more details about the surgery and potential needs that might come up. I would have a total of three IVs: one in my wrist, one in my hand, and one in my foot. A catheter would also be used during the surgery. It was likely that I would need a blood transfusion at some point, so they would prepare for that. Throughout the surgery, every vital would be closely monitored, and my anesthesia team would be ready to address anything that came up. The goal was clear: safety at all times.

My mom asked when they could expect me to wake up from the anesthesia. The nurse explained that it would depend on how my body reacted to the combination of surgery and anesthesia. Given the extent of the procedure and the amount of anesthesia I'd be receiving, they wouldn't be surprised if I didn't wake up until the day after surgery.

As always, there was a lot of information to absorb. But I found comfort in the way the nurse, who wouldn't even be in the surgery herself, spoke to us. She shared all the details with such confidence, as if the logistics of a surgery like this were routine and straightforward. Her calm assurance made it clear that, in her eyes, I was in the best hands possible.

After the nurse finished explaining the surgery details, my mom had some follow-up questions about the process and logistics. As they talked, I began to think about the anesthesiologist I had during my first surgery. He had taken such great care of my family and me, and I couldn't help but wish we could have him again. When the moment came, I spoke up and asked the nurse if she knew who the anesthesiologist for my surgery would be.

Just after I asked, the very anesthesiologist I had been thinking about walked in. He was just stopping by to say hello, but I couldn't resist asking him if he would be my anesthesiologist again for this surgery. He smiled and said he didn't think so but assured us that he would be one of the best anesthesiologists they had. He went on to say that she was much more talented than he was and that we were in great hands. Hearing him speak so highly of her was incredibly comforting. His respect for her confirmed the nurse's words that I was in good hands. And, as it turned out, even more comfort was on the way.

Before he left, he asked my mom and me if we would like him to pray over the surgery and the team that would be taking care of me. We were more than happy to agree, and he bowed his head and began to pray. The sincerity of his prayer brought even more comfort than his praise for his colleague.

One Last Weekend

The weekend arrived, and I had a couple of goals. The first was to finish school for the semester, and the second was to rest before the big day.

I had wrapped up most of my classes, except for my online science class, and there was still a lot to finish before surgery. I was taking chemistry that year, and to be honest, I struggled with it the entire semester. Trying to complete the last quarter of the course in just a couple of days was no fun. A scientific mind was definitely not one of the gifts God had given me. Thankfully, my school allowed me to retake tests as many times as needed, which turned out to be a huge blessing because I had to retake quite a few tests in that class. I remember asking Mrs. Morris to reopen my test about every 30 minutes over those two days. It was actually kind of comical because she was on vacation at the time, releasing those tests from a beach chair!

Relaxing in those final days before surgery was critical. I did everything I could to ease my mind and keep it as calm as possible before facing such a life-altering brain surgery. I dug out my coloring books and spent hours in them, letting the simple act of coloring help clear my thoughts. I also took naps whenever I could and watched a lot of funny movies.

I started reading the book of Psalms right after I found out about the surgery. Psalms is filled with praise for God and His unwavering faithfulness, and I felt that immersing myself in those words would be mentally beneficial in the month leading up to surgery.

Not only did I read through Psalms, but I also read other scriptures again and again, meditating on them all. Philippians 4:6-7 became a constant meditation for me, and I must have asked God for peace a thousand times during that month. I leaned heavily on these scriptures. While my anxiety was more manageable, it was far from gone, and the unknown still loomed. There were so many possibilities—scars, disabilities, things I couldn't even predict.

Only God knew what the outcome would be. Despite all that, I kept holding on to His peace. Thankfully, He provided it in abundance, and deep down, I knew that the surgery had a purpose. No matter what happened, everything would be OK.

The day before surgery had finally arrived. I woke up feeling a mix of anxiety and an unexpected sense of peace. It was strange but comforting at the same time. The first thing I did that morning was spend some quiet time. To me, it felt like one of my last chances to really sit with God before everything changed. I prayed over the surgery and what would follow. It was a moment to connect deeply with Him and bring my fears and hopes to the surface. This is the passage I read that day:

I cried out to God to hear me.
When I was in distress, I sought the Lord;
at night I stretched out untiring hands,
and I would not be comforted.
I remembered you, God, and I groaned;
I meditated, and my spirit grew faint.
You kept my eyes from closing;
I was too troubled to speak.
I thought about the former days,
the years of long ago;
I remembered my songs in the night.
My heart meditated and my spirit asked:
"Will the Lord reject forever?
Will he never show his favor again?
Has his unfailing love vanished forever?

Has his promise failed for all time?
Has God forgotten to be merciful?
Has he in anger withheld his compassion?"
Then I thought, "To this I will appeal:
the years when the Most High stretched out his right hand.
I will remember the deeds of the Lord;
yes, I will remember your miracles of long ago.
I will consider all your works
and meditate on all your mighty deeds."
Your ways, God, are holy.
What god is as great as our God?
You are the God who performs miracles;
you display your power among the peoples.
With your mighty arm you redeemed your people,
the descendants of Jacob and Joseph.
The waters saw you, God,
the waters saw you and writhed;
the very depths were convulsed.
The clouds poured down water,
the heavens resounded with thunder;
your arrows flashed back and forth.
Your thunder was heard in the whirlwind,
your lightning lit up the world;
the earth trembled and quaked.
Your path led through the sea,
your way through the mighty waters,
though your footprints were not seen.

You led your people like a flock
by the hand of Moses and Aaron that morning.
Psalm 77

Before that morning, I hadn't read Psalm 77. It just happened to be the next Psalm on the list. I had no idea what I would be reading, but I don't believe it was a coincidence that this was the passage I turned to the day before surgery. It felt like it mirrored what my soul had been through over the past two and a half months—the emotions and thoughts that were stirring inside me that morning. There were many times during those months when I would cry out to God, hoping He would take my pain away. And when I didn't receive an immediate answer, I would feel discouraged. Almost every time this happened, I'd slip back into the doubt that had existed even before I was diagnosed with cancer.

What's crazy is that almost every time, God showed up at exactly the right moment, making it clear that His hands were on me. He did this in so many ways—by placing a prayer warrior in our lives or leading me to the perfect scripture to read (like He had just done, once again). God reminded me of His miracles, His power in relationships, and His will to redeem what was broken. As I looked back on my journal entry from that day, it was obvious that I was in awe. Honestly, I'm still at a loss for words about how He worked during that time. After reading the scripture, I wrote down a prayer. It ended up being the final written prayer before surgery:

"God, thank you for this day! Tomorrow is my surgery, and I know you will be with me. Lord, I pray that you give me peace today and tomorrow. I pray you guide the surgeon and his team to get my tumor out. Lord, I have some goals that I would like to accomplish after surgery. I pray that you guide me to complete them. Thank you! Amen...

- I want to start drumming as soon as possible after surgery
- Drum at church by the fall
- Drum on the weekend
- Drum at C3 Conference
- Receive an A average in school
- Return to school my junior year
- Finish driver's ed by my next (16th) B-day
- Get a driver's license by 17

After writing these goals, I closed my journal and took what was probably one of the deepest breaths I had ever taken.

I spent most of that afternoon wrapping up the last tests in my chemistry class and soaking up time with my family. Austin, Brittany (the cousin who had come to see me at the hospital), my aunt, uncle, and grandparents were all coming over that evening for dinner. We were gathering not just to eat but to celebrate what we believed God was going to do in the surgery ahead.

As I was working through one of the final chemistry tests, my cousin Austin arrived. Once he got settled, he was eager to play some video games with me. But I still had that test to finish, and it was giving me a serious challenge. I couldn't seem to pass it. So, desperate times call for desperate measures, right? (Haha!) Austin, who had gone to college to pursue a degree in chemical engineering, tried to recall all the chemistry he could remember, and together, we somehow managed to pass the test. And just like that, I was finally done with chemistry!

We spent the rest of the afternoon hanging out, and as the rest of my family arrived, I felt the weight of their love and support in such a tangible way. My Uncle Tony had even taken off work so he and my aunt could be there with us on surgery day. My grandparents were praying over the surgery and telling everyone they knew about it, rallying more prayer around me. Both of my cousins had dropped their own plans and traveled miles to visit me throughout the fall.

We gathered together as a family and prayed for God to work miracles beyond our wildest imaginations in the surgery. But I'm confident we weren't the only ones praying. There were prayer warriors everywhere, lifting us up. I mention this not to boast, but to highlight and emphasize the incredible power of prayer. At the dinner table that night, my family was comforted by the prayers from those warriors.

After dinner was over, my cousins, aunt, uncle, and grandparents said their goodbyes and gave their last words of encouragement. Then they went to my grandmother's house to get some sleep before the next day. Oma was in from out of town and would spend the night. We took the rest of the evening to relax as a family.

That night, before I went to sleep, I prayed fervently. I told God all that was going through my mind. I praised Him for showing up in so many ways throughout the fall. I even referenced the "Red Sea" story again to underscore my awe at His power and what I believed He was capable of. I also laid out my worries before Him.

Most importantly, I did one of the hardest things I could do with the unknown ahead: I surrendered to God's plans for whatever was to come.

Much prayer was filled with the hope of healing, the kind we had believed God was capable of. God had plans and a purpose for what I was going through. I found out that fall, though, that His plans and timing were outside of ours.

The purpose of the chemo, for example, was to shrink and possibly destroy the tumor. My family and our prayer warriors prayed with confidence, believing God could make that happen. Some even prayed for the tumor to be gone entirely after the chemo. But when the results came in, the tumor hadn't shrunk one bit. If you remember, during that one check-up with my oncologist, he shared the potential complication of a decimated tumor. If the chemo had shrunk it too much, there would have just been a shell of dead cells left behind, and the doctors would have faced the tough decision of whether surgery was still necessary. In a way, the fact that the tumor didn't shrink turned out to be a blessing in disguise. It made the next steps clear—surgery was absolutely the next form of treatment, and my team knew what they were dealing with.

Ultimately, God knew the best solution to my sickness, and I had to trust that He would carry it out in His way and in His timing. The best-case scenario, in my mind, was for the tumor to be removed with minimal side effects. But I also knew there was a possibility that this might not be His plan. I needed to surrender to whatever His plan was for the surgery because, deep down, I trusted that whatever He had in store was the best.

So, I prayed for healing that night. I pleaded with God to save me from the threatening disease in my brain, but I also gave Him complete control. I put all the trust I had in His plan for the surgery, knowing that whatever His will was, it would be the best. After I finished praying, I lay still, trying to sleep, when suddenly, these words came to mind out of nowhere: "Your faith has healed you."

Over and over again, those words repeated in my mind. As I felt them come forth, my thoughts turned to Jesus in the Bible. I thought of those moments when Jesus told the people who came to Him in faith that they were healed because of their faith. They were healed and carried on with life.

One of these stories is found in Luke 8. In this story, a woman who had suffered from bleeding for twelve years touched the edge of Jesus' cloak in faith. The Bible says that "immediately her bleeding stopped." It also mentions that when she touched Jesus, He asked the crowd near them who had done so. The woman rose and explained why she touched Him. Jesus responded, "Daughter, your faith has healed you. Go in peace."

This was one of many times when Jesus said, "Your faith has healed you" in the New Testament. When I felt those words after praying, I hoped that my faith would lead to healing as well.

The next morning, my parents woke me up at about 4:30. Our bags were packed, so I only needed to get ready. I grabbed my favorite pillow, a blanket, my phone, and earbuds. We made a final run-through of the things I was taking to the hospital before heading to the car.

As I was heading out, I passed my grandmother, who was already awake and ready for the day. She and my sister would be coming to the hospital once surgery had begun. I gave her a big hug. As I pulled away, my head came close to hers, and she whispered her trademark phrase: "Grab that bull by the horns and kick butt!"

It was "go time," and I was ready to follow through with my grandmother's request!

We hopped into the car and headed toward the hospital. I put my earbuds in and meditated and prayed the whole way there. My nerves were sky-high, but a peace that transcended all my understanding was still present.

We arrived at the hospital, and as soon as my dad turned off the van, he reached for my mom's and my hands. We bowed our heads for prayer. My dad, as he had since the moment I first got off the MRI table, spoke with confidence in God. He voiced what we all felt—that we were giving control to God and declaring our trust in His plans, no matter what lay ahead. We finished with a heartfelt "Amen!" and then, as a family, we walked into the hospital.

Upon arriving at the surgery check-in, my mom dove into filling out a mound of paperwork while I sat on the couch beside her. The waiting room felt quiet, and all I could do was recite Philippians 4:6-7 over and over to myself. As I repeated those words, my soul called on God's name with reverence.

After what felt like an eternity, a nurse came in and brought my parents and me to surgery prep. They took my vitals and then hooked me up to the first IV after I had laid down. My parents and I engaged in small talk, and both of them were already receiving texts of encouragement.

At about 6:00, my anesthesiologist appeared through the door and introduced herself. She gave us her plan for the surgery and mentioned the possible blood transfusion that her team was ready for. She asked if we had any questions, and then she headed toward the operating room to get ready.

Moments later, Dr. Honeycutt (my brain surgeon) appeared through the door. I was surprised by his appearance. He was wearing a sweatsuit and was completely relaxed. I thought he would be in scrubs, with a surgeon cap on, and be nervous even though he had done this before. However, he looked as if he was going to lounge around for the day. I guess his ability to stay relaxed was a good thing, though.

Once again, he explained the details of the surgery that was about to take place. It would be a craniotomy, where he would reach my tumor by going through the center of my brain. He reassured us that he would be very careful, making sure the tumor wasn't penetrating the brain stem. Once he located the tumor, he would use a specialized tool to carefully suck it out. After the surgery, I would be taken to recovery and then moved to the ICU, which is where they expected me to wake up.

He again asked if we had any questions, and I responded, "You said you are confident, right?"

"Yes, I am," he replied.

That was all I needed to hear, and I told him I was ready to go.

After he checked with my parents to see if they had any questions (as far as I can remember, they didn't), he gave us a nod and then asked us the only question he had, "Would y'all like me to pray before we start?"

As with my first brain surgery, we answered with a yes when Dr. Honeycutt asked if he could pray. Just like the prayer months earlier, it brought a profound sense of peace to our hearts. I knew God was moving.

Dr. Honeycutt said his goodbyes and left the room. It was time for my parents to give their final words of encouragement and tell me goodbye. The reality of the moment settled in: the surgery was truly in God's hands now. He was the only one who could guide the team through it, and I had complete faith that He would. Whatever the outcome, I knew there would be a purpose in it, and that purpose would refine my faith in ways nothing else could. I surrendered it all over to God one last time. Within the next minute, the nurse administered the relaxing medicine, and the world around me began to blur. It was time to enter the fire.

CHAPTER TEN

I woke up to a nurse calling my name. It seemed like it was only five seconds earlier that I was in surgery prep and saying goodbye to my parents. When the nurse realized I was conscious, she said, "Christian, you're out of surgery! You are in the ICU."

I was happy to be out of surgery. I was even more excited that I was in recovery and could talk to the nurse. Even in my barely awake state, I wondered what the result of the surgery was. I called out to the nurse, who was standing by my bed. "Did he get the tumor? Is it gone?"

"Yes," she answered, "I believe he got all of it!"

Instantly, peace overcame me, and I could do nothing but rejoice. I was barely coherent and couldn't tell what side effects were present, but that didn't matter. All I cared about was the fact that my tumor was gone!

Finally, the nurse came over and told me my parents were there, but I was too tired to open my eyes. Then, I felt some people next to me and heard my mom's voice say, "Hey, Bubba!"

It felt amazing to hear and understand her voice, especially since we didn't know if that would happen. "Bubba" had been a nickname my family had called me for as long as I could remember, and it's how my mom always greeted me. Hearing it again brought me comfort at that moment, and I was so grateful for the chance to hear it. I joyfully replied, "Hi, Mama." She started crying tears of joy, and those two words still mean more than we can ever put into words.

Hearing my response and realizing that my speech was intact, my mom exclaimed, "Your tumor is gone!"

With what little energy I had left, I raised my hand and flashed a "rock on" sign, signifying our battle cry of "Rock on, Christian." It just felt right to throw up the sign and show my excitement.

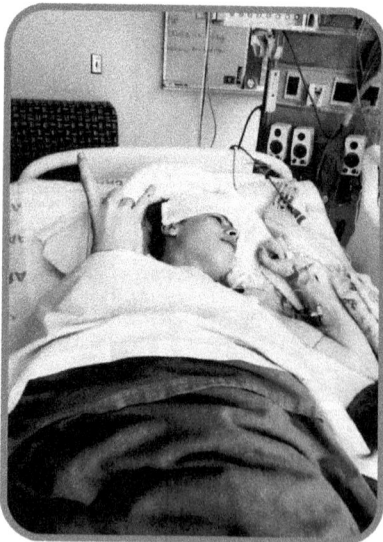

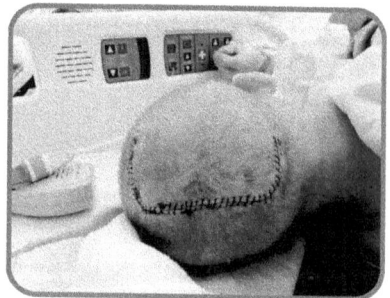

As my mom kept talking about the surgery results, she said my stitches looked like those on a baseball, and my scar was the shape of a big C.

Some might see this and think of the name Christian, but to me, it reminds me of "Christ." He saved my life through this surgery. A curveball was thrown my way, and God stepped up to the plate in my place, hitting it with power like no one else could.

My parents checked on how I was feeling and congratulated me on the miracle that had just happened. I had just woken up, so we didn't know what side effects might show up yet. But the fact that the surgery was a success and I was able to talk was a huge blessing and a miracle. It's hard to explain how excited I felt, knowing the cancerous tumor was no longer in my head.

My journey was not over, though. I needed to recover from surgery, which was a challenge itself, and radiation would follow soon after that. It wouldn't be long before the side effects from surgery became clear, and more were expected to hit from radiation. I was ecstatic and thankful for God's guidance during surgery, but the journey was not over.

Over the next hours, the immediate side effects from the surgery kicked in. I was on strong painkillers, so the pain was manageable, but nausea started to hit hard. Every time I tried to turn my head, I ended up vomiting. I was still exhausted, and my eyes stayed closed. When I tried to open them, they didn't seem ready for the light. So, I had to rely on my hearing to figure out what was going on around me.

That night proved to be more challenging than anticipated. One might expect that after undergoing invasive surgery, with anesthesia still lingering and the body aided by painkillers, rest would come easily. Yet, I found myself waking every couple of hours. Somewhere in the ICU, a light flickered, and its glow seemed to trick my mind into believing it was morning. I remember being so happy when morning finally came and then wanting to sleep because I was so tired (Haha!).

A nurse entered the room and casually informed my mother that the doctor had scheduled a routine MRI to assess how my brain was recovering. Though the words were directed at my mom, I overheard them, and immediately, I wanted to protest. I was tired and didn't have the emotional strength to endure an MRI, but Dr. Honeycutt was resolute about it.

Memories of my first MRI began to resurface. All I could recall were the deafening sounds of the machine and the unsettling dread of potential bad news. I lacked the energy and mental strength to meditate on verses like Philippians 4:6-7. The only solution was to ease the tension in my mind with morphine. Before long, I was wheeled into the room with the MRI machine, where I was carefully transferred onto the table. They draped a warm blanket over me and played soft music in an attempt to keep me comfortable. The procedure passed in a blur, and before I knew it, I was being gently lifted onto a gurney for transport.

Amidst the haze of everything, there was a bit of good news. We learned that my vitals had stabilized enough for me to be moved into a regular room. It had only been 17 hours since surgery, yet here I was, ready to be moved to a regular room. The doctors had originally anticipated that I'd need to stay in the ICU for at least two days, but that expectation was shattered. Another "impossible" had been swept away by the Lord's hand, a reminder that His power can defy all odds.

Transferring to my hospital room was a quick process, and it brought the "excitement" of being lifted again with it. My best friend's dad and mom met us in my room, and though I couldn't make much sense of it at the moment (morphine and hydrocodone), I am so thankful that they came to check on me.

I slept for the majority of that afternoon. But at some point, the results from the MRI came back and showed that my brain truly was tumor-free! My family and I rejoiced again! By now, all of us were exhausted. My parents had spent the last 48 hours praying fervently and putting every ounce of faith they had in God. The surgery felt like five seconds to me, but it must have felt like five years to them. I can't imagine what went through their minds during those seven hours. They were facing one of the biggest unknowns of their lives. Would their son's dangerous tumor be removed through surgery? The exhaustion from facing the unknown with courage was worth it. God worked a miracle in a surgery that could have turned out very differently, and their son was healed!

That night was tough for me. The morphine from earlier in the day was still in my system, which made sleep, well... interesting. According to protocol, the nurses came in throughout the night to check my vitals. In between their visits, I managed to sleep, but I kept having the same recurring dream. I found myself in the movie

Coming to America, playing Eddie Murphy's role as the Prince. For those who haven't seen the movie, Eddie's character gets tired of the constant royal treatment and decides to move to America to live a more normal life.

There's a scene in the movie where the royal attendants are always by Eddie Murphy's side, constantly asking if he needs anything. That scene kept replaying in my mind every time I slept between the nurses' check-ins. Eventually, the dream and reality started to blur. I would wake up to the nurses asking if I needed anything, and at that moment, I pictured the royal attendants from the movie. To make it even more surreal, my feet were touching the end of the bed, and my covers were all tangled up. I was uncomfortable and just plain tired of being treated like royalty by my "attendants."

After the dream hit again, I woke up and shouted for my mom. She rushed over and asked what was wrong. In my discomfort, I blurted out, "I want a bigger bed, fewer sheets, and for everyone to stop treating me like a king!"

My mom was able to fulfill my first two requests, but the third puzzled her. Before long, my bed was extended, my sheets were straightened, and I was settled in comfortably. I had to settle for being "treated like a king," though, as my nurses still needed to check on me regularly.

It must have been the next morning when I woke up to find my mom and one of her close friends, Mrs. Shala, in the room. My mom had stepped out to make some oatmeal for me, and I tried to sit up to get ready to eat. However, as soon as I did, my head spun, and the nausea hit hard, making it clear that it wasn't such a great idea. I immediately became sick, prompting my mom to rush for a bucket while Mrs. Shala grabbed towels, both of them calling for the nurse. We still aren't sure what caused it, but I believe it was just my brain adjusting to the movement again.

The "incident" from that morning, combined with the lingering anesthesia in my system, left me completely exhausted. I remember drifting in and out of sleep, keeping my eyes closed even when I was awake. I don't recall much else from that day, except for one visit that meant everything to me.

At some point in the afternoon, I was lying on my side when I heard someone walk into the room. I heard what sounded like my mom standing up from her chair to greet the visitor. Then, I heard him ask, "Is he awake?"

"Yes. He just likes to lay with his eyes closed, but he can hear you," replied my mom.

As soon as I heard those words, I knew exactly who had come to visit. It was Derric, the head worship leader at my church, the same person who had texted my mom while we were in the emergency room after the first MRI. My body, still weak and drained of energy, didn't show it, but inside, I was filled with excitement. It meant the world to me that Derric had taken the time to come visit.

I soon felt a tap on my shoulder. Derric had come over to my bed and was greeting me. He told me he didn't want to disturb my rest but was so relieved that the surgery had gone well. He then sat down in a chair next to my mom, and they started talking as quietly as they could. Derric shared how inspired he and the church had been watching our family fight through everything over the past few months. He suggested that creating a video about our story would be a powerful way to share our journey of faith and resilience with others.

I heard my mom respond with excitement and gratitude as if she wholeheartedly accepted my "proposal." She agreed that everything that had happened over the past few months had come together to tell an incredible story of God's miraculous healing. I'm not sure if they realized I was awake or not, but from my bed, I agreed enthusiastically (inside my head)!

I was blown away by what God had done through the surgery. But just a couple of days later, He gave my family and me an incredible opportunity to share His faithfulness and healing power with many people. As strange as it might sound, I realized that something bigger and more significant was happening than just my healing.

The third day was one of the toughest in my recovery. At some point that morning, a physical therapist came in to help me start walking again. The nausea had finally settled, and I could move my head without feeling sick, so I was eager to get up and walk with ease. But that wasn't the reality at all.

As I tried to stand, I felt incredibly weak and off-balance. My nurse and dad had to help me stay upright. The first goal was to walk to the bathroom door and back to my bed, but I could barely manage it. The lack of strength was frustrating, and I couldn't help but get upset. I was struggling to walk just three days after major brain surgery. Oh, the irony!

It was clear that my brain was far from fully recovered. It still needed more rest and time to heal, and it deserved that time. Sharp instruments had just navigated through its cavities, and now my brain was trying to regain control over basic functions like movement, balance, and walking. I was healed, but I had to be patient and allow my brain the time it needed to fully recover.

The problem was I hadn't fully accepted that reality. I wanted to recover quickly and kept pushing myself to do things like sit up and walk again, even though my body wasn't ready. It took some wise words from an important medical professional, who by now was a close friend, to snap me back to reality and remind me to slow down.

Amid all the excitement surrounding my first steps since surgery, my nurse practitioner walked into the room. I'm not sure if someone called her or if it was just God's perfect timing (maybe both), but she immediately saw that I was struggling. She walked over to my bed and told me exactly what I needed to hear at that moment: "Christian, you need to allow yourself to be sick. You had an invasive brain surgery three days ago! Do you know that most kids who go through this surgery are still trying to wake up three days after it, much less walk? You have been miraculously healed, and that is great! However, your body still needs time to recover and be sick. Don't be down on yourself, but rejoice in your healing and give it time to rest and recover!"

I needed to hear those words from Mandy, my nurse practitioner. She reminded me to be thankful for the simple fact that I was healed, not to mention awake and still myself. Even though I was struggling to walk at that moment, I knew it would come back to me. My body just needed more rest, and I finally accepted that I had to let it happen.

I slept through most of the afternoon. Later, my surgeon came by to check on my progress. After going over my vitals and chatting with me for a bit, he said, "Well, if you can stay in this condition through tomorrow morning, and you promise to try and walk a lap in the hall, I will probably send you home tomorrow afternoon."

"What," responded my mom, excited and shocked, "He is only four days out of surgery."

Dr. Honeycutt nodded and responded, "I know. I don't necessarily want to send him home, but medically, I have no reason to keep him."

My mom and I were stunned. I couldn't believe I was going home just four days after surgery. Before all this, the expectation had been that I'd be in the hospital for at least two weeks to recover. But once again, God had worked beyond our understanding, smashing another expectation and shortening the recovery time in a way that only He could.

My dad usually went home in the evenings to be with my sister during those days. But it didn't take long for the news to reach him, and he was just as stunned as we were.

That evening, my goal was to rest as much as possible so my body could gain strength and have enough energy to meet Dr. Honeycutt's requirements the next day. On top of that, Mandy's words still lingered in my mind. I needed to take it easy, both physically and mentally, to give my body the best chance to keep healing.

Expectations, Hope, and God's Provision

I'd like to take a moment to reflect on our expectations and God's plans. Throughout this journey, it's become clear that healing and restoration haven't unfolded in the way my family and I anticipated or wished.

There's a difference between anticipating something and simply wishing for it. Expecting something to happen carries a greater sense of confidence. It's about waiting for it to come to fruition. On the other hand, hope introduces a level of uncertainty. When we expect something, we're certain it will happen, even if we don't know exactly when or how. But when we hope, there's a recognition that the timing, method, or even the possibility of it happening might be out of our control. Hope, in that sense, requires a deeper dependence on the source that will make it happen.

It's interesting how the Bible consistently encourages Christians to place their expectations and hope in God. It teaches us to anticipate that God will do great things and that He wants us to trust in Him to fulfill those promises. One of the most well-known verses is Jeremiah 29:11, but to truly understand its significance, it's important to consider the full context of the passage.

Jeremiah 29:10-13: "This is what the Lord says: 'When seventy years are completed for Babylon, I will come to you and fulfill my good promise to bring you back to this place. For I know the plans

I have for you,' declares the Lord, 'plans to prosper you and not to harm you, plans to give you hope and a future. Then you will call on me and come and pray to me, and I will listen to you. You will seek me and find me when you seek me with all your heart.'"

The broader passage shows that God's desire was for Israel to seek Him. I believe the reason God wants us to have hope is that it brings us to a place where we rely on Him. There are likely several reasons for this. First, I think it's because God loves us and wants to provide for our needs. Second, I believe it's because God understands our inability to see into the future and the uncertainty that comes with that.

Throughout my journey, I've seen how God operates in unexpected ways. Even though His method of healing turned out to be the best, our limited perspective made it hard to see how one situation could set the stage for a miracle in another. Only God could guide us through the plan He had for my healing.

Returning Home and Overcoming Expectations

Both of my parents were filled with joy and gratitude toward God. They prayed fervently for my healing but never imagined that just four days after surgery, I would be able to walk a full lap around the hall. We had expected a much slower recovery, but God had other plans, allowing my healing to progress far faster than even my surgeon had predicted.

Once Dr. Honeycutt heard the news, he came to do one final check of my vitals. After reviewing them, they were still strong enough for me to be cleared for release. Once the discharge paperwork was completed, I'd be able to go home!

I was beyond excited to be released and couldn't wait to go home! The discharge paperwork took a couple of hours to process, which felt like an eternity. But even after all that time, the excitement still hadn't worn off. We were all celebrating and praising God for His miraculous healing.

Once my mom and dad gathered their things, we were ready to go. My dad went downstairs to bring the van up to the hospital entrance while my mom and the nurses helped me into a wheelchair (I'd done enough walking for one day!). We made our way downstairs and out to the front. As we approached the entrance, the sunlight coming through the windows was too bright for my eyes. So, my mom grabbed a pair of sunglasses and put them on me. Suddenly, I was rolling out of the hospital in style! (Haha!)

I woke up the next morning feeling excited. That day, I was finally going to be able to go home to my dogs, sister, and grandmother. All I had to do was walk a lap around the floor I was staying on. My muscles were still weak, but I was determined to make it happen.

Deciding to walk wasn't as simple as just getting up and going for it. For my safety, I needed a physical therapist to accompany me. She would be there to support me if my legs gave out and help me regain my balance if I started to wobble. Plus, I had just opened my eyes that day, and they were still adjusting to the light and movement around me. I also had some slight double vision, which was expected. The therapist acted as an extra set of eyes, guiding me through the walk and ensuring I stayed steady.

Later that morning, the therapist came in, signaling that it was time for my walk. I was determined to finish the lap. She helped me get out of bed and secured a special belt around my waist, which had a loop at the back so she could support me as I walked. Once everything was set, we slowly made our way to the door and out into the hall. One step at a time, with her assistance, I made my way down the hallway. As I walked, I could feel my balance starting to return, but I knew better than to get cocky. I kept relying on the therapist for support.

As I rounded the corner and got closer to my room, my dad met us with his camera, walking beside me. My mom was waiting by the entryway, doing her best to hold back tears. I had done it. I had taken steps again and completed an entire lap around the hallway.

CHAPTER ELEVEN

It took about a week for me to feel strong enough to go back to school. I felt good, but I was still a bit tired, and I was adjusting to some side effects with my vision from the surgery. I had double vision, and my right eye was turning outward. Both were expected and would be fixed with surgery later. Sometimes, my right eye would drift to the side when I looked at things from a certain angle. However, it wasn't a big problem and didn't stop me from getting most things done.

An occupational therapist from the hospital set up occupational and physical therapy for me. Thankfully, after assessing me, she realized I only needed physical therapy. My fine motor skills were recovering better than expected, so I didn't need both therapies, which was a relief. Even though I was recovering well, I still had to take it easy. My parents and I decided to keep my schedule as light as possible. Physical therapy was going to help me with things that were affected by the surgery, like my balance.

With physical therapy set up, I spent the rest of the week getting stronger and getting ready to go back to school. I was nervous about it, though. I wasn't sure how well I'd be able to learn or write because of the surgery's effects.

School resumed the following week, and Mrs. Morris came for our first session of the semester. I remember her greeting me at the door with a lot of excitement. She had been praying with other warriors for my surgery to be a success.

After some small talk, we got to work. We planned to take things slow, but I still had a health test to finish. Mrs. Morris said it was mostly common sense and that she could help if I needed it. I took the test and then moved on to the rest of the day's work.

It was good to see Mrs. Morris again. She has a signature phrase she likes to say, and she said it that day: "Upward and onward!" It felt just right for the moment. I was tumor-free, and it was time to move forward, starting with getting back to school and getting ready for radiation treatment.

Moving on From Surgery

The original plan after surgery had been to do full brain and spine radiation, followed by six more rounds of chemo. However, one day in the hospital, Dr. Murray got the pathology report for my resected tumor and discovered that the chemo hadn't affected it at all. Because of this, he felt that doing six more rounds of chemo would be pointless. He decided that radiation would be the last treatment and mentioned they were considering just targeting the tumor bed in my brain with radiation.

This was a big decision. The MRIs after surgery showed no signs of the tumor, and my blood was clear of cancer. But that didn't mean there weren't any cancer cells still lingering in my brain. So, my oncology team had to decide whether my whole brain was at risk or just the tumor bed. My oncologist planned to meet with his team and other specialists from across the country, including one at St. Jude Children's Research Hospital, to figure out the best treatment approach.

One might wonder, "Why not just play it safe and do radiation on the whole brain?" The reason was that, aside from surgery, radiation was expected to cause the most lasting side effects. It could lead to issues with processing and cognitive function, and radiation to the entire brain could affect my ability to produce a range of important hormones. So, the goal of only treating the tumor bed was to avoid some of those tougher side effects and make life after treatment a bit easier.

It took a couple of weeks for them to decide on the details of the radiation, so I tried to focus on recovering and keeping up with school. Now and then, I'd sneak off to my room to play the drums. Of course, there was no way to play drums secretly, and I was still pretty weak. I even had to relearn some drumbeats. But it felt like therapy. A big part of drumming is hand-eye coordination, so practicing helped me get that skill back. Plus, drumming had always been my way to relieve stress. I told myself it was just another part of the healing process.

I think it was around Thursday of that week when an amazing opportunity arose. Derric called my mom to talk about the video my church wanted to make about our family. Besides showing it during the weekend services, Derric suggested I could come out on stage and play a song with our church's worship team, Fellowship Creative, as the drummer. We'd play "Lead Me," a song they had written for people experiencing the storms of life.

When my mom asked if I wanted to do that, I'm pretty sure I jumped for the first time since surgery. Not only would we get to share our family's story, but my dream of playing drums on the weekend (a goal I had written down before surgery) was about to come true. I was beyond excited! Right away, I grabbed the link to the song and started practicing.

A lot of great things were happening, but I still tried to rest and take it easy. The heavy anesthesia from the surgery was still lingering in my body, and I needed sleep. My appetite was also still low. I remember taking afternoons to relax and watch TV. Since my mom was still off work, she was taking care of me while my dad went back to work. Our afternoon tradition became watching The Ellen Show after my post-lunch nap. It was nice to spend that time with her, and I cherished those moments together.

The next week, physical therapy started, and we also had an appointment to hear the doctor's decision. I remember my therapist coming to the house and doing some tests to check my balance and muscle strength. One of the first things she asked me to do was a sit-up. I thought, "Only one sit-up? Pffft... no problem." So, I lay down on my back and tried to do the sit-up.

But when I tried, something surprising happened… I couldn't do it. For a couple of minutes, I struggled and failed miserably! My therapist and my family all laughed, and it was a moment of the Lord humbling me. My therapist explained that I shouldn't feel embarrassed because the surgery had affected my muscles in ways I didn't expect. It was pretty common for patients to experience this a couple of weeks after surgery.

After doing some balance tests, my therapist decided we needed to focus on muscle and balance exercises over the next few weeks. The goal was for me to regain the ability to do a sit-up and improve my balance, even on one leg.

I continued with school, and Ms. Bernard came back for our first math session since the surgery. Even though I had a lot going on, we were behind and needed to catch up. That meant I'd have more math homework than usual over the next couple of weeks. Like with Mrs. Morris, I was happy to see Ms. Bernard again. Amid the grueling geometry problems, we also caught up on life.

I enjoyed the conversations with both of my teachers. From the start, they made it a point to do more than just teach me. They also wanted to be there for my family and me. They genuinely cared about us, and it felt so good to be able to talk with them about life in between assignments.

Getting back into school was an adjustment, and I did struggle with stamina. Thankfully, I had the support I needed to keep moving forward. Little by little, my strength and appetite started to come back. At this point, life was all about pacing myself, and we were grateful every day that I was even able to resume normal activities so soon after surgery.

Sharing Our Story

At some point between starting therapy and getting back to school, my church's team came to our house to film the video of our story. They filmed my parents together first, then my sister and me separately. My parents were asked to start at the beginning and share everything they could remember. The crew also told them not to hold back any emotions while telling the story.

Watching my parents recall everything that had happened over the past few months was breathtaking. Their words brought back all the fear and uncertainty we had faced, the physical and emotional pain, and the unexpected healing we couldn't fully grasp. One moment that stood out was when my dad talked about me asking if I was going to die and how his heart sank when I asked that question. It was hard not to feel the weight of his words as I listened. But the best part was hearing them praise God at the end of the story. A victory had taken place in our battle, and all they could do was look up to God in gratitude.

After my parents, it was Lauren's turn. She's the kind of person who speaks clearly and joyfully, without any drama, and always brings light into our lives, even during tough times. But that didn't mean things were easy for her. As we listened to her share her side of the story, it hit us that this was a trial for her, too. The support and wisdom she showed were truly remarkable. I remember her talking about praying to God before the surgery, begging Him to be with us and the medical team that day. She also spoke about trusting in God's ability to heal. She found strength in Philippians 4:13 and relied on it, knowing that God's power would carry us through.

I went last. Listening to my family's testimonies was amazing. I was, and still am, so thankful for them. It was clear that they fought just as hard as I did and that our story wasn't about their glory or mine. It was all for God's glory. The theme of our story was God's faithfulness in healing and restoring those who call on Him.

The week of January 25th finally arrived, and I was so excited. The weekend was going to be the debut of my family's story at church. That Wednesday, Fellowship Creative released their album (which included the song I would be playing on stage) and held an album release concert. They played through the entire album, and my family was there to worship and praise God with everyone. Afterward, we stayed behind to film me playing the drums for the video. I was in my happy place, hitting the drums to the different beats. Joy oozed out of every hit!

Before we knew it, the video was finished, and the long-awaited weekend arrived. At the time, my church had a Saturday service in addition to the Sunday ones. I had been practicing nonstop for the past couple of weeks, wanting both the video and the song to go as smoothly as possible. My family and I hadn't seen any of the video yet. All we knew was that the team was making the final cuts and edits. We had no idea how we would react to seeing it. But we did know that every emotion tied to our trial was sure to wash over us and the audience when it aired.

I got to church around noon that day for rehearsal, and the nerves were already starting, even though it hadn't begun yet. I walked backstage as the band finished setting up. Before practice started, they decided to grab lunch, and soon the place was empty. One of my worship leaders walked through and invited me to go to Starbucks with him. I agreed, and we headed out for some coffee. Even though it was just a five-minute ride, he filled that time with nothing but encouraging words, helping to calm my nerves.

Soon, we were back at the church, and rehearsal started. The first few times we ran through the song went smoothly, and the band sounded great. It was time for the run-throughs.

The team finished the video, and I remember watching from backstage. As it played, I went on an emotional rollercoaster. The scene where my dad talked about me asking if I was going to die, the part with my sister's words of wisdom, and the one with my mom reflecting on seeing me for the first time after surgery - all of those made the final cut. I was brought to tears as each of those moments unfolded. Then, a scene came up where I talked about the gift that each day on this earth is, and that hit me hard, too.

I started to remember the advice my nurse practitioner had given me just a few weeks before we got the news about the tumor not shrinking. She had encouraged me, with all her heart, to make the most of every day because no day is promised. Gratitude for God's faithfulness over the past few months and His gift of more time through the tumor's removal filled my mind. But there was also something inside me telling me that my healing wasn't just for my own benefit.

We finished the remaining run-throughs, and it was only a matter of time before the service began. We went out to the atrium to greet guests, and I found my family to let them know what they were about to experience during the service. We shared a moment of joy, and then it was time to head backstage and get ready for the service.

Once we entered backstage, our head worship leader gathered everyone together, and we prayed over the entire service. He prayed that everything would go smoothly and that we would all look to God as we fulfilled our different roles. The service was going to be packed with worship, my family's story, and a powerful message. In his prayer, he asked God to work through all of these moments so that someone in the congregation would turn to Him that night. When the prayer ended, it was officially time for the service to begin.

As I watched the worship set from backstage, my nerves came rushing back. I tried to focus on worshiping God and not let any distractions take control of my thoughts. Just like before, I surrendered to God and reminded myself that He was the reason everything had unfolded the way it had. He was the One deserving of all the praise for my healing and for the chance my family had to share our story.

Before long, the worship set was over, and they moved on to announcements. That was my cue to head over to the back of the riser. There was a set of stairs that would take me up to the drum set, and I sat down on them, quietly preparing. I remember praying over the next ten minutes of the service.

After our worship leader finished the announcements, the drummer from the worship set came down the stairs and gave me a fist bump. It was time to take my place for the song. As the video started to play, I sat down at the drum kit and made a couple of adjustments. The video continued, and all the emotions from before came flooding back. My family was sitting in the first few rows, and I could see my mom, who had brought tissues for the video. As high as I was on the riser, I could make out her wiping away tears as she listened to the story of the past few months. I'm pretty sure I saw my dad wipe away a few tears, too.

As the video came to a close, I tried to calm myself and prepare for the "swell" out of the video. When the teleprompter started counting down the last ten seconds, I lightly swelled on the cymbals, and the band followed me (no pressure). After a crescendo, we came back down to settle the moment. Our head worship leader then introduced me to the crowd, followed by an introduction to the song and its story. He dedicated it to my family and to anyone in the audience going through a trial. Then, the metronome in my in-ears kicked in, and the song began!

I remember taking the song beat by beat, each measure feeling like it stretched into a minute. Yet, somehow, the song flew by so quickly. As we played through the chorus, I embraced the lyrics. The words at the end of the song still sit in my heart today: "Father lead me, Spirit lead me, Jesus lead me." Those words captured the essence of everything I had experienced over the past few months. In both the times I turned to God and the times I turned away from Him, He was still the One leading me through the storm.

176

Restoration came when I finally surrendered to Him, but He had been with me through it all. The journey wasn't over, though.

CHAPTER TWELVE

I walked off the stage feeling vibrant and on top of the world. On my way to the green room, I hugged almost everyone I passed. The next two services on Sunday felt just as great. It was an awesome weekend!

In the days after, we had an appointment with my oncologist to find out what kind of radiation they had decided on. The options were either full brain and spine radiation, which came with a lot of side effects, or treating just the tumor bed, which would have only a few minor effects. I felt some anxiety leading up to the appointment, but through God's guidance, my surgery went better than any of us expected. In a way, it felt like I had dodged a bullet, or more like God made the bullet miss me. Full brain and spine radiation would be the next bullet heading toward me, and with it, certain side effects like processing issues and hormone deficiencies, almost in the same way that eye issues were promised from surgery.

But I trusted that God would guide us to what was best for me, and my family did, too. In the final hours before the appointment, we tried to fight the anxiety by remembering how God had carried us through everything so far. We held onto hope that even if full brain and spine radiation was the choice, God would protect my brain from the side effects.

We arrived at the hospital that morning, sticking to our tradition of praying before our visit. After checking in on the oncology floor, we sat down to wait. I glanced at my mom, and she mouthed "I love you" to me. My dad was sitting next to her, quietly praying. Soon, a nurse came out and called us back for a vital check. After that, she led us to the conference room to wait for Dr. Murray and Mandy.

Eventually, Dr. Murray and Mandy walked in. As Dr. Murray greeted us, they sat down across the table. I suddenly felt a sense of déjà vu, like I was back at the diagnosis appointment from the previous September.

Originally, the plan after surgery was to do full brain and spine radiation, followed by six more rounds of chemo. But one day, while in the hospital, Dr. Murray got the pathology report for my resected tumor and discovered that the chemo hadn't even affected it. Because of this, he felt that going through six more rounds of chemo would be pointless. He then said that radiation would be the final treatment and mentioned they were considering only targeting the tumor bed in my brain with radiation.

I remember feeling disappointed when they decided to go with full brain and spine radiation. Even though I knew deep down it was the right call, especially with a tumor doctors didn't fully understand, I knew we had to take every precaution to make sure it didn't come back.

Dr. Murray explained the radiation plan in detail. He told us that the treatment wouldn't be done at the hospital because a new type of radiation was now available. I would be going to the Texas Center for Proton Therapy in Irving, and my treatment would be managed by Dr. Mangona, a radiation oncologist. The plan would require daily visits to the clinic for six weeks. Like chemo, radiation could lower my white blood cell count and cause nausea, so I'd have weekly check-ins with Dr. Mangona to monitor those issues. When he finished explaining everything, Dr. Murray wished us good luck and said he'd see us in a couple of months after the treatment.

More Treatment and Affirmation

My first appointment with Dr. Mangona was just a few days after the one with Dr. Murray. That morning, we headed to the radiation center. As soon as we walked in, we were greeted by a familiar face. Cara was a child life specialist I had met at the hospital. It turned out that just a couple of weeks earlier, she had transferred from Cook Children's Hospital to the Texas Center for Proton Therapy.

When I saw Cara, a sense of peace washed over me. She would be my child life specialist throughout the radiation process. Little did we know, she would end up becoming like another Mandy to me.

Soon, Dr. Mangona came out and introduced himself. He was very kind, and from the moment he spoke, I could tell he was someone I could trust. He was easy to talk to and had a calming presence. He then led us to a room with a patient table, some chairs, a desk, and a computer. We all sat down, ready to hear the details of the plan.

Dr. Mangona started by telling us about the team at the center. They had spent years researching and carefully selecting the best candidates to form the team. It was made up of top radiologists from all over the country, and he reassured us that we were in great hands. He also mentioned that the credentials of the team were one of the main reasons he and his family decided to move from Detroit and join the center.

Once again, a feeling of peace settled over me. My family and I exchanged glances, knowing deep down that God had brought the right people into our journey. We hadn't even started radiation yet, let alone heard all the details, but we felt confident that God had already taken care of the next few weeks.

After introducing the team, Dr. Mangona began explaining proton therapy. He shared that radiation had been around for a while, but it was originally only in the form of Photon therapy. With Photon therapy, a radiation beam was directed at the area needing treatment. While it could target tumors, scientists hadn't been able to control it perfectly, meaning it often affected surrounding organs. For example, if someone had a tumor in their spine, the photon ray wouldn't just hit the tumor. It would pass through and impact organs like the liver and digestive system.

With proton therapy, they can now target the exact area that needs treatment and have the ray stop once it's done in that area. So, in the spine example, the ray could stop at the edge of the spine, preventing it from passing through and damaging other organs. And, unlike photon therapy, they can control how much of the radiation is delivered to each part of the body. As Dr. Mangona would probably agree, proton therapy was a breakthrough in cancer treatment, and this center had only been open for a few months.

If you do the math, this center had opened just about a month and a half after my diagnosis appointment. If radiation had been the first treatment option, I would've had to go to the next closest proton therapy center, which was in Houston, four hours away. Seeing the timing of it all, I couldn't help but recognize it as a blessing from God.

After explaining proton therapy, Dr. Mangona went over my specific treatment plan. He pulled up my MRI from the day after surgery, along with a color-coded diagram of my brain. He pointed out that each color represented a different amount of radiation. In the full brain and spine treatment, some areas of my brain and spine would receive higher doses, measured in grays, than others. The center of my brain, where my tumor was, would naturally get the highest dose of radiation.

At one point during his explanation, Dr. Mangona stopped mid-sentence. He looked at me, then glanced back at the MRI image. Turning toward my parents, he said, "It's not every day that a patient emerges from a major surgery with an MRI scan this clear, nor is it typical for them to experience minimal side effects while retaining their personality. Such a combination is extremely rare. I must say, your son is a medical miracle."

I think my parents and I just looked at each other and smiled. It was more confirmation that God had truly worked a miracle through the surgery. I imagine it's pretty rare for a doctor to call something a miracle. They're trained to know the range of possibilities, so not much is likely to surprise them. But that is how magnificent God is.

Dr. Mangona continued, outlining the logistics of the radiation. For the first four weeks, they would treat the entire brain and spine. After that, they would focus solely on the tumor bed for the final two weeks. No matter which area was being treated, though, I would need to go to the proton center every weekday.

As for side effects, Dr. Mangona explained that the short-term ones included nausea, headaches, hair loss, and fatigue. Hair loss and fatigue were just part of the process, but he was confident that they could manage the nausea and headaches with medication. The long-term side effects, however, were more concerning. Radiation would affect my brain's pituitary gland, which produces hormones, because it hadn't fully developed yet. On top of that, processing issues were expected to come up after treatment, which could make things like learning or problem-solving more difficult. However, Dr. Mangona was optimistic that, even though these side effects were expected, the precision of proton therapy would make their impact less severe.

Dr. Mangona was an optimistic person, and his positivity was evident throughout the entire appointment. This was exactly what we needed as we braced ourselves for radiation. We knew the next few weeks would be tough, and there was still a lot of uncertainty ahead. But over the past months, God had shown us that His control was something we could trust. That didn't mean challenges wouldn't come after radiation, but we learned that God, in His sovereignty, didn't keep us from facing difficulties. Instead, He stayed right by our side, carrying us through each one. With that in mind, we shared Dr. Mangona's optimism, knowing that no matter what lay ahead, God would lead us through it.

We wrapped up by going over the next couple of weeks before radiation started. Dr. Mangona explained that I'd need to come in for a CAT scan and an MRI before treatment. The scans would allow the radiation team to project them onto the radiation table to target the beams properly. They would also create a mask to strap my head to the table, ensuring I stayed secure during treatment. Once that was all set, we could begin the radiation.

When I heard I'd need another MRI, even though it wasn't to check if the tumor was gone, a wave of anxiety hit me. It had been six or seven months since the MRI that first found the tumor, but apparently, that wasn't enough time. In that moment, I realized that no matter the purpose of the MRI, it always stirred up a lot of emotions as I walked through that hallway.

I didn't want to go through another MRI. But the truth was, the radiation needed to be accurate. I knew I'd have to put on a brave face and push through it. My meditation strategies were still helpful, and I'd be relying on them to get through.

After the consultation, Cara came back in and showed me a video that explained what radiation would be like. It was a cartoon, set in a room that looked almost like a cave, with a table in the center. A girl came into the room and lay on the table, and technicians adjusted her and put on her mask. Once everything was set, the technicians walked out, and you could hear the sound of a doorbell. Then the radiation beam started and treated her for a few minutes. Afterward, the technicians returned and unhooked the mask, and the girl got up to go back to her grandma. Although it was made for younger kids, the video gave me a clear idea of what radiation would involve. It was reassuring to know a bit more about the process before starting. After the video, our consultation wrapped up. They took some baseline vitals before radiation began, and then we were on our way.

An Amazing Opportunity

It must have been toward the end of that week or the beginning of the next when we decided to push back my radiation treatment. Every year, my church holds a big conference that attracts our members, other churches, and church planters from all over the country. It's a huge event, and since my mom had gone back to work, she would be working at it. My dad and I also wanted to attend. The only problem was that the radiation was scheduled to start during the same week as the conference. So, we called Dr. Mangona to ask if it would be possible to move everything back a week. To our surprise, he agreed, and my dad and I were able to attend the conference.

I was so excited to be healthy enough to attend the conference. Physical therapy was going well, and my stamina was slowly improving after surgery, so it didn't feel like a huge risk. My mom and I started brainstorming possible ways I could volunteer. One day, just before the conference, my mom came home from work and suggested I serve at the booth for our church's worship team. She thought it would be a good fit since they'd have stools at the booth for me to sit on, and they'd be promoting and selling the team's new album. That sounded perfect to me. Not only would I get to help out at the conference, but I'd also get to work with some of the people I was closest to at the church, without overexerting myself. I gladly accepted her idea.

The day of the conference finally arrived, and I woke up feeling ecstatic to be part of it. I went to church with my mom, who had to get there early. We helped out with the final preparations, and soon, the first day of the conference was underway. In between each session, I sat at the booth and helped the worship team promote the new CD. We also got to attend the sessions, where incredible speakers from all over the world shared powerful messages.

Spending those final days before radiation at the conference was truly special. One of the main themes throughout the event was celebrating God and what He was doing through the church. I'd heard my whole life that the church is not a building but a people. Those few days were the perfect example of that definition. People from different churches, all across the U.S. and the world, came together. Even though they gathered in different buildings on the weekends, they were all united in praising the same God for His faithfulness and for making a relationship with Him possible. My family and I shared that same perspective, and God certainly deserved all the praise that week for so many reasons.

The night before the last day of the conference, my mom got a call from one of our church's worship leaders, Aaron Weits. She answered the phone and started talking to him. After a few minutes, she turned to me and said, "Christian, they want to show our video at C3 (the conference) and want to know if you want to play Lead Me afterward!"

I think I almost fainted when I heard that! I don't remember exactly how I reacted, but I know I was ecstatic and accepted with gratitude. My mom confirmed with Aaron that I'd love to play the next morning and hung up the phone. Then came the real challenge—trying to get some sleep that night so I'd have enough energy for the big day. It was going to start super early since I needed to be at rehearsal by 6:15.

It wouldn't surprise me if I spent the whole night dreaming about playing at the conference the next day. Around 5:00 the next morning, my mom came in and woke me up. After I had gotten ready, we headed to the church. We pulled up to the stage-side door on the outside of the building, and I made my way into the backstage area. All the band members and worship leaders were still trying to wake up. They chatted while drinking coffee.

Our worship leader, Derric, appeared backstage and greeted my mom and me enthusiastically. He asked if I was ready, and even though I was nervous, my excitement outweighed it. He reassured my mom that they'd take good care of me. Then, he introduced me to the drummer they had brought in for the conference. He was such a nice guy and shared how excited he was for the morning, too.

Soon, the run-through began. The service would kick off with one of the songs from the new album, followed by announcements, where they'd introduce our story. Then, it would be time for the video. As before, that would be my cue to climb onto the drum riser and get ready for the song. After the video, we'd perform the song, then end with a powerful swell into the message. Rehearsal went smoothly, and I was feeling ready to play.

The session I was part of would be the second one that morning. During the first session, I went to help out at the booth. Before we knew it, the first session was over, and it was finally time to fulfill one of the biggest dreams I'd had up to that point. On top of that, people from all around the country were about to hear a testimony of God's faithfulness. Of course, they hadn't already heard plenty of those at the conference!

My mom was busy at her post, and my dad had a work appointment, so he couldn't be there. I didn't get to hug my mom before going on, but she would make it to the audience by the time the video started. I went backstage, where the team gathered to pray over the service and the story. As soon as the word "amen" was spoken, everyone hurried to their positions. A few moments later, the first few bars of the song kicked in, and the worship team began leading the audience in worship.

The opening song of the service was called "Jesus Our Hope." It felt so fitting because He had truly been our family's hope throughout the last few months. That's not to say we didn't have doubts. I've shared some of those doubts with you already. But Jesus was bigger than those doubts and broke through them. Hope, at its core, is the desire for something to happen. Through every setback, pause, or breakthrough, our desire for healing and deliverance from death never wavered. We held onto the truth that Jesus had already defeated death. Despite the doubts, we put our faith in His authority over it all. We had hope that, even if my life on earth wasn't spared, I would ultimately be in heaven, free from pain, and with Jesus for eternity.

The song ended, and the announcements started. I was standing at the bottom steps of the big riser, stretching and praying. I praised God for giving me another chance to share our story and fulfill a dream. I asked Him to work through the video and the song so that people would be inspired to face their struggles and turn to Him in everything.

The announcements wrapped up, and the lights in the auditorium dimmed for the video. As it started, I began walking up the riser. The drummer passed me as he walked down, giving me a quick "bro hug" and offering some words of encouragement. When I reached the top of the stairs, I was greeted by the sight of an enormous crowd. There was just enough light to see that about 3,500 to 4,000 people were out there. While I couldn't make out anyone beyond the first couple of rows, I knew my mom was somewhere in the balcony, among the church staff.

I adjusted everything I needed to while the video played, then sat back and watched it with the audience. About twenty seconds before it ended, I got my sticks ready and kept an eye on the band leader as he guided us through the transition. On his count, I started to build with the band. The lights brightened, and we went into some big swells. As we played, Derric introduced me. Between hits, I tried to give the audience a small wave. You might wonder if seeing such a huge crowd was nerve-racking, but honestly, it would've been if I could see them. The drum cage caused a glare from the lights, so I could barely make out anyone beyond the first few rows. I just pretended I was back in my room, playing as usual.

Just like a couple of weekends before, Derric praised God for His faithfulness through the storm. Then, we swelled into the song. It was a bit of a whirlwind. I remember playing and feeling pure joy, but it all ended just as quickly as it had started. We powered through each verse and chorus, worshiping together as a band. A dream and goal of mine had come true. It was hard to believe that only a month after major brain surgery, I was playing drums for an audience of thousands. Moments later, we hit a big crash-out as the song came to a close. The lights faded to black, and I walked off the riser with the rest of the band.

As soon as the service ended, I found my mom, and we embraced with so much joy. I think we called or texted my dad to let him know everything went great. After that, I went back to the booth to help out. Throughout the morning, people from all over came up to the booth to share in the joy. They expressed their gratitude to God for His healing and how inspiring our story had been. We rejoiced together, over and over, about what God had already done through our video, and about how my dream of playing the drums in front of so many people had come true.

The week of the conference flew by. Along with everything related to the video, we also had to prepare for radiation. I went to the proton center to get my mask made, which was a quick and easy process. I also had the MRI and CT scan done. The MRI ended up being much easier than I expected. It only took about twenty minutes.

CHAPTER THIRTEEN

M y first radiation treatment was on a Monday. We got to the proton center in the morning, and Cara greeted us at the door. They gave me an ID to use for check-in so they could start my treatment. After that, Cara sat down with us in the lobby while we waited for my appointment. We chatted and got to know each other a bit more. There was a lot of laughter, which would become common in the weeks ahead. The light conversation helped calm my nerves.

Soon, a radiation therapist came through a door, signaling it was time. My mom gave me a big hug, and then Cara and I followed the therapist down a confusing hallway. We turned into a section with several curtains, like dressing room doorways. The therapist led me into one of the empty rooms and handed me a gown. Like with an MRI, I had to remove my outer clothes and change into the gown.

Once I was changed, I met the therapist and Cara in the hallway, and they led me back to the "cave." As we turned the corner, I saw a table suspended in the air, and above it was a huge cube-shaped object. Suddenly, the cube started spinning clockwise, moving from above the table and eventually landing on the ground. It was one of the coolest things I'd seen, but the room itself was so strange. On one side, it looked like something out of a Marvel movie with its twisting, cave-like section. On the other side, there was a more normal area with hardwood floors, cabinets, and counters.

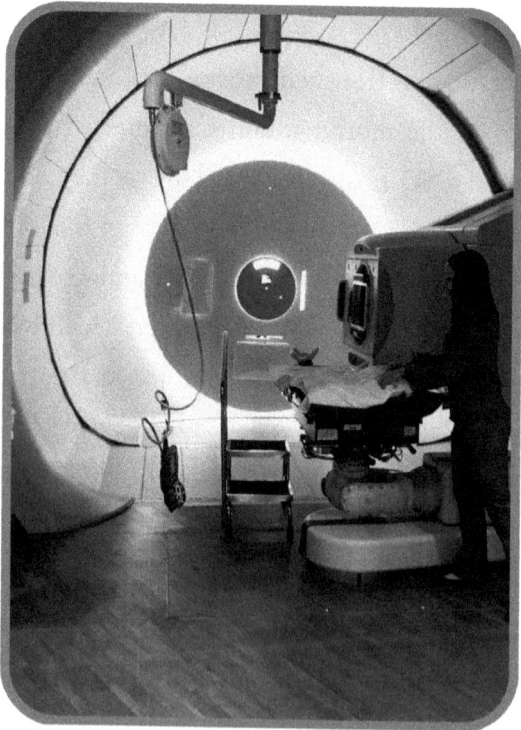

More therapists came in from a room just outside the cave and introduced themselves. They were friendly, but you could tell they were serious about their work. Cara told me she would stay with me during the appointment, except when the beam was on. At that point, she and the therapists would have to leave for safety reasons. This was comforting.

After they lowered the table, one of the therapists helped me onto it. They brought over my mask and placed it on me once I was settled. It was important that I not move once I was in position because even a small shift could mess up where the beam hit. For the next 30 minutes or so, they projected my MRI and CT scans onto the table, making small adjustments each time. To keep me from getting bored and moving, they played some music in the background. Eventually, they had me in the perfect position. A therapist came over to tell me they were going to start the beam. From a distance, I heard Cara wish me luck, and then I heard a doorbell.

I braced myself for what was coming, trying to focus on reciting the verse from Philippians and staying as still as possible. Suddenly, I heard a "poof" sound, but I didn't feel anything at first. About 30 seconds into the treatment, though, I started seeing blue flashing lights. That seemed odd, and then something else happened. A metallic smell filled the air, my body felt warm, and I started to feel dizzy. It was like the sensation someone might get after being electrocuted but without the pain. That awful feeling lasted about 15 seconds before it faded. Then another "poof" happened, followed by a doorbell. I wasn't sure what had just happened, but I knew it hadn't been pleasant.

A therapist popped in and told me they were about to start the next beam for my lower spine. I braced myself even more, expecting another strange feeling. But this time, as the beam went on, I didn't feel anything at all. It seemed to last the same amount of time as the first one, and soon, another doorbell and "poof" sound followed. Then a technician came in and said they were going to treat my upper spine and then be done. Once again, I heard a doorbell and "poof." When the treatment ended, the therapists came back and took off my mask. I slowly sat up and let out a big "Whew!" I still couldn't quite figure out the strange sensations I'd just experienced.

Cara led me back to my changing room and waited patiently while I changed. Once I was ready, we walked back into the lobby where my mom was waiting. We shared another hug and then went to see Dr. Mangona for a quick check-up to see how I was feeling and how the first treatment went. I felt fine overall, and despite the weird sensation, the first day wasn't too bad. I didn't bring up the sensation to Dr. Mangona, though. I'm not sure why—I think I just wanted to see if it happened again. But I couldn't deny that what I'd felt during the treatment was uncomfortable.

After the appointment, my mom and I took a photo by the sign outside to commemorate the occasion. We were both tired and ready to relax for the rest of the night.

Walking Through Radiation

The next day, my dad took me for my second radiation treatment. Cara was in the lobby to greet us again. I checked in with my badge and then sat down near my dad and Cara. When the therapist came out to take me back, my dad wished me luck by saying, "Have a nice flight!" I think I chuckled at that, but honestly, it kind of made sense because I was suspended in the air on the table. So, in a way, I was flying. Over time, this would become my dad's signature phrase before each treatment, and it became something I looked forward to hearing.

My second session was almost identical to the first. It took them about the same amount of time to adjust me before starting the beam. Another thing that mirrored the previous treatment was the weird and awful sensation that I felt during the beam that treated my brain. After this treatment, I knew I had to tell Dr. Mangona about it.

During an appointment with Dr. Mangona that week, I decided to mention the flashing blue lights and metallic smell I'd experienced. I wasn't sure how he'd react, and I could see how it might sound a little strange. But when I described it to him, he didn't seem puzzled at all. After thinking for a moment, Dr. Mangona explained that the beam hits a nerve in full brain radiation, which can cause a weird smell for a small number of patients. He said the blue flashing lights were new, though. My first thought was, "Thank goodness I'm not crazy," and the second was, "Of course I have to be in the minority or a 'special case' with everything related to cancer!" (Haha!)

Knowing that other people were experiencing the weird sensation was encouraging, but the problem wasn't solved yet. I asked Dr. Mangona if there was anything we could do about it, and he paused to think for a moment. After a bit, he said he would need to look into it further.

The next day, when I arrived for my treatment, the therapist mentioned that Dr. Mangona suggested we try spraying my mask before the "brain beam" to help deter the smell. I was all for it. So, right before that beam, one of the therapists sprayed a mint scent on my mask. As the treatment started, I prayed the peppermint spray would help. But about 15 seconds in, the blue lights and metallic smell returned. The peppermint was still there, but the metallic smell was as strong as ever.

Unfortunately, there wasn't much more they could do about the sensation. Dr. Mangona wasn't concerned about the nerve being hit, either. So, I realized I was just going to have to power through the rest of the full brain treatment as best as I could.

Over the next week or so, the sensation made each treatment really tough. I couldn't get used to it, and I started moving during the beam. This was a big issue because even a small movement could mess with the accuracy of the beam. My therapists tried to help me stop, but I felt awful. After every treatment, I'd get off the table and immediately ask them how much I had moved. Even when I tried my hardest not to, the sensation was so bad that all I could do was flinch. That little movement was enough to throw off the beam.

One day, when I arrived for treatment, one of my favorite therapists greeted me. She told me that they had been trying to figure out how to solve the problem of movement and came up with an idea. This was to switch the order of the beams so that the last one would be for the brain. To make sure, they checked with Dr. Mangona, and he said that changing the order would be fine. At first, I wasn't thrilled about the idea. The thought of building up to that awful sensation in the last beam felt daunting. But I was willing to give it a try, so that's what we did. Surprisingly, it worked well. The sensation was still terrible, but since my head was locked in place by the mask, I didn't move it when I flinched. Plus, I was able to stay completely still during the other beams leading up to it.

I'm so grateful for the therapists who helped me get through the toughest part of radiation. Their patience and creativity made the full brain and spine treatments much easier than they could have been. With their support, I was able to power through that challenging part of the radiation.

It's not that I didn't ask God to take away the sensation. I truly believed He could lessen my nerves' sensitivity. But for some reason, He didn't. Why, I'm not sure. Maybe this small trial in the middle of radiation was meant to make me stronger. Or perhaps the purpose of having to push through the treatment with that sensation was to help me become more flexible, something I've struggled with my whole life.

Reminder of the Inevitable

When I think about the challenge I faced during radiation, I'm reminded of characters in the Bible. Take Job, for example. Despite living a successful life, he had to face the destruction of everything he knew—his wealth, his family, and his health. The Bible describes him as a man who was "blameless and upright; he feared God and shunned evil". Job's wealth was immense and included 7,000 sheep, 3,000 camels, 500 yokes of oxen, and a large number of servants. He had everything anyone could desire. Yet, despite his success and faith, he faced a deep struggle. But God had a purpose in it. After Job remained faithful through the disaster, he was rewarded in ways he couldn't have imagined. Scripture says that God gave him twice the splendor he had before.

My point in sharing this story isn't that I think I'll be rewarded with riches for going through that awful sensation. Instead, I believe that even during the high points of life, trials still come. No matter when they arise, they always have a purpose. In my case, God had just removed my tumor through a miraculous surgery, and my family and I celebrated that every day. But that didn't mean life was done throwing curveballs my way. The sensation I dealt with during radiation was just one of them.

Another Light at the End of the Tunnel

For the last two weeks of treatment, they focused only on the area where my tumor had been. Dr. Mangona predicted that the sensation I had been feeling would go away because that nerve wouldn't be affected anymore. Thankfully, he was right! In the first treatment of the tumor bed, I didn't feel a thing. It was such a relief! I knew getting through these next two weeks was going to be much easier.

The last two weeks of radiation flew by. I tried to appreciate my time at the proton center and the people who made it easier. Every day I came in for treatment, Cara and I would find something to laugh about. That was just the nature of our relationship. I can't remember a time when I was with Cara that she wasn't smiling. She's one of those people whose smile can light up a room. Even on the tough days, when that sensation got to me, Cara always found a way to make me smile. I have no doubt she was yet another person God placed in my family's life at just the right time.

Before we knew it, the final day of radiation arrived. This day meant more than just finishing the treatments. Dr. Murray had consulted with pediatric oncologists across the country to get their input on which type of radiation would be best. After considering the professional opinions of his colleagues and reviewing my diagnosis again, Dr. Murray concluded that full brain and spine radiation was the best option. It was the safest choice, as they didn't want to risk missing any cancer cells that might be lingering in my brain or spine. They also decided that continuing with chemo after radiation wouldn't be effective since it didn't target the tumor directly.

So, not only was it the last day of radiation, but it was also the last day of cancer treatment altogether! My mom told me that morning she was going to meet my dad and me at the proton center afterward to celebrate this huge milestone. I couldn't believe it. Today, I would finally be able to say I was done with cancer treatment. What a blessing! I was so excited to celebrate the end of this journey with my parents.

The final session of radiation went by quickly. The therapists were ready as soon as I changed, and the setup didn't take as long as it had before. Before I knew it, the final doorbell rang, and the beam started. I tried to keep my excitement in check and stay as still as possible. After a couple of minutes, I heard one last "poof" sound, and the therapists came in to help me off the table for the last time.

One of the therapists walked me to my final appointment with Dr. Mangona. When we entered the room, my parents were already there and immediately got up to hug me. Not long after, Dr. Mangona came in, did a quick check of my vitals, and sat down to ask how I was feeling. The answer was "amazing." Despite dealing with some fatigue, I had very few headaches, and my nausea was under control. Even if I was experiencing these symptoms, though, the joy I had would have numbed them.

n. Dr. Mangona reviewed the treatment that I underwent one last time. He said that after overseeing the process and keeping track of how the treatment was affecting me, he was optimistic about my future. It was too early to tell whether I would go to college or how the impeding processing issues would affect me, but he was hopeful that they would not hinder my ability to live a normal life. This was great news to hear!

When the appointment ended, my parents and I headed toward the lobby, eager to get home and move forward with life. As we approached the door that led into the lobby, my mom pulled her phone out of her purse. It seemed a little odd at the time, but as soon as we opened the door, I figured out why. On the other side of the door was a lobby full of family and friends, my whole support team. The staff and Dr. Mangona, both of my grandmothers and grandfather, my best friend and his family, and my sister and dad were all there. As I walked through the door, my best friend made his way over to me, and we embraced in a hug I will remember forever.

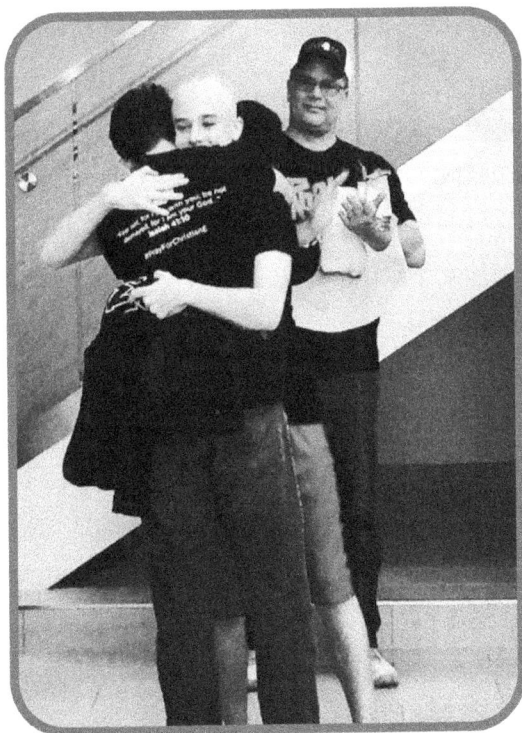

We had a big celebration in that lobby. After my parents introduced everyone to Dr. Mangona and his staff, it was time for the special moment that every patient at the Texas Proton Center gets to experience when they finish treatment. I got to hit a huge gong, and the victorious ring it made was such a powerful sound. It felt like a perfect way to mark the end of this chapter.

We continued talking for a while, enjoying the celebration. At one point, my dad noticed a lady sitting by herself in one of the chairs in the lobby. She looked sad and lost. My dad went over to her and struck up a conversation. After a few minutes, he learned that she had a daughter who was currently undergoing radiation. They were just at the beginning of their journey, not at the end like I was. There was so much uncertainty ahead of them. After hearing all of this, my dad came back to the rest of us and suggested that we pray over her. My best friend's dad is a pastor, so it felt right for him to lead the prayer. We walked over to the woman and asked if we could pray for her daughter. She nodded, and we gathered in a circle, holding hands as we prayed for her and her family. It felt like the most meaningful way we could offer support at that moment.

That prayer might have been one of the most meaningful parts of the celebration. We were done fighting a deadly disease, but there were, and still are, many others who have to fight for their lives every day. That moment was also one of the first times I realized that our story had a purpose beyond just our own healing. It could help and encourage others. When facing a fatal illness, it's easy to feel lost and alone. But after that day, I knew we would have more chances to pray for and uplift others, and I was determined to make sure we did just that moving forward.

Moving Toward the End of Treatment

Over the next month or so, I focused on finishing school. I was caught up in most of my classes, but math was a different story. In both semesters, it felt like Ms. Brenard and I just couldn't catch up to the rest of the class. When she came over to help, we had to work hard and fast, pushing through multiple assignments at once to get back on track.

One day, when she was over, we were looking at the work ahead, and she sighed. I asked what was wrong, and she said, "I just don't know how we are going to get this done."

When she said this, the thought of having to repeat geometry hit me hard. Looking at the pile of work in front of us, the stress overwhelmed me. Before I knew it, tears were streaming down my face like a river, and I couldn't stop crying. Ms. Brenard was speechless, clearly shocked, and trying to figure out how to comfort me. Within seconds, my mom rushed into the dining room from the back, and both of them did their best to calm me as I cried uncontrollably.

Ms. Brenard offered words of encouragement to both my mom and me. She acknowledged that there was a lot of work to catch up on but assured us that we would find a way to make it happen. She said she would talk to the administrators and my teacher to see if we could skip a couple of units to make it more manageable. After hugging me, she stood up from the table. As soon as our session ended, she went straight to my school to see what could be done about the math work.

This moment was one of the first signs that my processing skills weren't functioning as they once had. I had cried before, but never because of stress alone. At that moment, the stress triggered an uncontrollable wave of tears. If I were to paint a picture of what was going on in my head, it would be like a dam on the verge of bursting. The pressure built up until the walls couldn't hold it anymore, and in a matter of seconds, everything just broke through. Over the following months, there would be many more moments like this one.

By the time our next session came around, Ms. Brenard had worked everything out with the school and my math teacher. Given the extenuating circumstances, they decided to cut one of the units from the curriculum. This took a huge weight off both of us. There was still plenty of work to be done, but we felt much more confident that we'd be able to finish it all in time.

Physical therapy was another part of my routine that continued over the next month. My therapist came over once a week for a session, and we focused on exercises to improve my balance, like heel-to-toe walking and standing on one leg. She became another friend to me during that time, and we'd talk about everything as we went through our walks. It made the sessions feel less like therapy and more like just another part of my week where I could connect with someone. Talking to her during the exercises made them a lot less boring, and the sessions felt a lot more manageable. It wasn't long before my therapist felt that my strength and balance had improved enough. In our last session, she asked me to do a sit-up, and this time, it was a piece of cake, so different from the first one!

As April came to a close, my final MRI was fast approaching. If it came back clear, they would officially declare me in remission. Naturally, anxiety started to build up as the day drew closer. The weight of this MRI felt heavier than much of what had happened up to that point. I clung to Philippians 4:6-7 during that time, meditating on it regularly. On the weekend before my MRI, my best friend and I celebrated his birthday by taking shooting lessons from some Marines. This might have been a more fun way to de-stress before a big event. We had so much fun and learned a lot from those men.

The MRI soon started, along with *The Blind Side's* first couple of scenes. I meditated diligently while watching the main character in the movie get introduced to his new school.

Not long after that, some familiar words popped into my mind: "It will be OK." Just hearing those words brought a sense of calm, and I let them sink in as I continued meditating. With the contrast injected and only about fifteen minutes left in the MRI, I focused even more on those words, quietly thanking God for His faithfulness. Finally, the MRI came to an end, and the tech came in to help me off the table.

We had some time between the MRI and the appointment, so my mom, dad, and I decided to grab lunch. We went to Torchy's, and I was excited because it would be my first time trying their tacos. I've got to say, it was a great choice. Afterward, we took a deep breath, braced ourselves, and headed back to the hospital.

The second we parked the van, my dad grabbed my mom's and my hands, and we bowed before the Lord. I don't remember the exact words of his prayer, but I do remember feeling my dad's deep confidence in God, who had been with us every step of the way throughout treatment and that morning. His prayer was full of trust in our Heavenly Father. When he finished with an "Amen!", we got out of the car, ready to head into what we hoped would be an appointment of triumph.

It didn't take us long to check in and make our way up to the fourth floor for our appointment. My mom grabbed the "how are you feeling" sheet to fill out while my dad and I sat down. Other than the butterflies in my stomach, I was feeling fine. The headaches and anxiety were at bay, so physically, there wasn't much for me to worry about.

I continued praying for peace as we sat there. Then, a nurse came through the door to call us back for the appointment. We went through the usual vitals and were escorted to the room where the results would be given. Out of all the appointments I had during those months, waiting for this one felt like the longest. I'm not sure how much time passed, but I must have meditated a hundred times, sitting next to my parents, trying to stay calm in that room.

I was in the middle of praying through the verses when, out of nowhere, my surgeon appeared through the door. My heart stopped for a moment, and I slowly looked up at him. He asked how we were doing, and I think my parents and I all nodded in response. My dad must have asked him how he was doing because he started talking about hunting ducks the previous weekend. It felt a little strange. Here we were, waiting for life-changing news, and he was casually telling duck-hunting stories. But in the middle of his tale, he paused, looked at us, and said, "Oh, and the scan is clear."

Immediately, my parents and I jumped out of our seats with cries of joy. My dad was punching the air and thanking God while my mom broke into tears.

We celebrated for a good five minutes while Dr. Honeycutt sat back and embraced the joy present before him. At some point, Dr. Murray entered the room during the celebration. He congratulated us and went straight into the final spiel of my journey through cancer treatment.

He walked us through a review of the planned treatment and what had happened. As he spoke, all the emotions from the first brain surgery, chemo, the final brain surgery, and radiation flooded my mind. We didn't mind hearing it all again, though, because it reminded us of God's faithfulness every step of the way through the battle with cancer.

I get emotional just remembering those moments. Words can't fully capture how grateful I am to God for His faithfulness. In that instant, it felt like I had exited the tunnel and stepped into the light I had seen from a distance when I discovered 1 Peter 1:6-7. And just as the verse predicted, God was glorified. Through His grace, I had been saved as a young boy. Through His grace, He pursued me in my doubt and showed me His presence in my life. Through His grace, He forgave me and stayed by my side when I turned away. Finally, through His grace, He healed me so I could testify to His miraculous power.

Once Dr. Murray finished, I felt like there was one thing left to do. In a way, my first big moment in this journey began with a prayer. Prayer had been a huge part of my strength and trust in God throughout this trial. So, it felt right to end this chapter by praying with both Dr. Honeycutt and Dr. Murray. I didn't hesitate to ask, and they were more than willing to join me in lifting our voices to God, praising and thanking Him for the miracle we were witnessing. When we finished and lifted our heads, three words echoed in my mind: "It is finished."

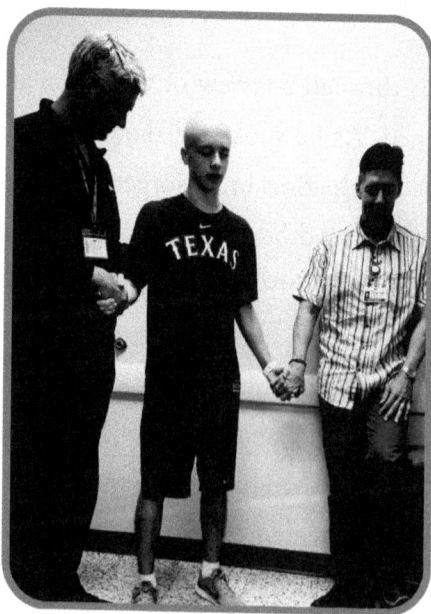

CHAPTER FOURTEEN

𝘐 t has been nine years since that glorious appointment, and we've continued to celebrate all the incredible ways God worked throughout my journey with cancer. For the rest of my life, I will praise God for carrying my family through the unthinkable. But my journey didn't stop when Dr. Honeycutt said, "Oh, and the scan is clear." Since then, I've navigated the recovery process, adapted to a new normal, and tried to reconcile the many questions that shaped my battle with cancer.

A Much-Needed Getaway

After my appointment, my family and I were exhausted. For the last nine months, we had been dealing with the physical and mental challenges of cancer treatment. It wasn't until we heard the news of remission that we could end "fight mode". As I started recovering, we needed a way to unwind from all the stress and anxiety. Luckily, we didn't have to look far. The end of treatment gave us the perfect chance to pick up where we had left off with my plans at Make-A-Wish.

I had brainstormed many times about what I wanted to do for my wish. This encouraged me because I had something to look forward to. As cancer took its toll, I felt like I should wish for something that my whole family could enjoy together. That's when the idea of a dream vacation in paradise came to me. I started thinking about going to Hawaii.

I will never forget that trip. From the moment we arrived, we knew it would be a vacation like no other. We were greeted with leis at the airport, welcomed to our hotel with gifts and a pass for its VIP lounge, and given a room with a balcony that overlooked the ocean. We were truly in paradise.

Over those few days, we were truly able to ease our minds and rest. We got to snorkel in the clear blue ocean, where I saw a fish that looked like cotton candy (I didn't even know those existed!). We swam with dolphins, zipped over the beautiful, lush island of Oahu, and even attended a luau. At the luau, the Polynesian people gave their special blessing to my family.

But out of everything, the best part was being in such a beautiful place with no stress. Make-A-Wish took care of all the details, and we were treated like royalty everywhere we went. All we had to do was relax and forget about everything we'd been through as a family. This trip was a much-needed reset and helped us recover from the effects of my fight with cancer.

Adapting to a New Normal

As amazing and refreshing as the trip to Hawaii was, nothing could prepare us for adjusting back to normal life. Honestly, I've come to believe that there's no such thing as going back to "normal." The cancer treatment was over, and I wasn't facing an immediate threat to my health anymore. But when I tried to pick up where I left off before cancer, my family and I noticed that I was different. How I thought and how I functioned had changed. The chronic side effects we'd been warned about were starting to show up. Now, nine years later, I'm still dealing with those effects, and they don't seem to be going away.

The first challenge I've faced is fatigue. During surgery, Dr. Honeycutt didn't just remove the tumor; he also had to take out my pineal gland. This gland's main job is to produce melatonin, which helps regulate sleep and our internal body clock. Without my pineal gland, I've had a hard time falling and staying asleep at night. As a result, I'm constantly low on energy, and the only way to recharge seems to be by taking naps during the day. But, of course, that's not always practical, and real life doesn't give us adults much time for naps.

Another side effect is processing issues. Dr. Mangona had warned me about this due to the radiation, but I didn't fully realize how much it would affect my life until treatment ended. These issues have created challenges that I deal with every single day. This includes disorientation. My brain processes completing tasks differently.

For example, if we're sitting in a booth at a restaurant and you ask me to grab a napkin, it's not as simple as just walking up and getting it. First, I have to stand up. Then I need to figure out where the counter with the napkin dispenser is and plan my route to it. If I pass someone and need to adjust my path, I have to find the counter again. Once I reach it, I need to spot the napkin dispenser among everything else on the counter and grab the napkin. Then, on my way back, I have to repeat the process.

It sounds like a lot just to get a napkin, right? But that's how my brain works through nearly every task I do. Each step has to be processed and mapped out in real time. Add in the disorientation, and daily tasks become a constant challenge.

Another challenge I've faced is losing control over my emotions. You might remember an incident during a homeschool session with Ms. Bernard when the stress of homework made me cry uncontrollably. Unfortunately, that wasn't a one-time thing. As time went on, we noticed that even the smallest things could set me off and cause me to burst into tears.

The cause of my emotional struggles wasn't a mystery, though. It was another side effect of my brain's processing issues. The areas responsible for processing emotions were damaged, which made it physically impossible to handle things like sadness, anger, or stress. It also affected my ability to process positive emotions like joy, gratitude, and love.

To this day, I still cry when I feel overwhelmed by any emotion. Is this a threat to my health? No. But it has made social interactions difficult, especially at work when stress triggers tears, and I end up making a scene. Over the years, I've worked with several counselors to cope with these emotional challenges. We've made progress, but it seems like I'll be battling this inability to process emotions for the rest of my life.

The lack of emotional control ties into another major challenge I've had to deal with: post-traumatic stress disorder (PTSD). PTSD is, unfortunately, common in our society, and according to the Mayo Clinic, its symptoms can include flashbacks, nightmares, severe anxiety, and intrusive thoughts about the traumatic event. I experience all of these, but the worst has been the chronic anxiety.

Over the years, I've worked with counselors to help me cope with the anxiety that comes with PTSD. Some days are better than others, but anxiety attacks are still a regular part of my life. When one hits, it feels like I can't breathe, and I have to rely on breathing exercises for a few minutes to get it back. On top of that, I meditate on verses like Philippians 4:6-7 and talk things through with someone to help calm myself down.

The truth is, beating cancer didn't bring me back to a "normal" life. The fatigue, processing issues, and PTSD showed up right after treatment and are battles I'll face for the rest of my life. I'll keep dealing with these challenges and learning how to cope with what my family calls a "new normal."

The Problem of Trials

The reality of this "new normal" and the challenges it brings serves as a reminder that surviving a tough disease didn't free me from facing more struggles. And I'm not alone in this. Every person faces trials throughout life until they move on from this world. This brings us back to the same questions that started this book: Why do we go through trials? How do we overcome them? And can any good come from them?

As I mentioned at the beginning, these questions often lead people to wonder how an all-powerful, loving God can exist alongside such tough trials.

If we look at my journey through treatment, it seems to point to the work of something, or someone, beyond myself. The way everything lined up so perfectly, with such personal care and timing, makes it hard for me to believe it was just some random force at work. With all my heart, I believe it was God who left His fingerprints on my healing and restoration.

When we look at the beauty, intricacies, and patterns in our universe, it's hard to believe that "chance" is the only cause behind it all. The idea of everything coming together by chance would itself be an astonishing miracle. There has to be something behind it, and that must be a powerful, personal being.

I don't think the existence of trials (and the evil that often leads to them) is enough to disprove the existence of God. However, I do think that suffering in this world challenges the idea of a God who is good, loving, and just in everything He allows. It's a tough question that we wrestle with.

So, what do we do with this problem? Is there any way to reconcile the immense pain that humans inevitably face and justify faith in a loving God?

Yes, I believe there is.

An Answer to the Problem

I have to admit I'll never have a perfect, all-encompassing answer to why God allows suffering in this life. But beyond my limited understanding, Scripture shows us a God who has good plans and is just in everything He allows. I've pointed to some of these passages in my story, and there are many more throughout the Bible. So, when searching for an answer to this problem, we have to remember these truths. And I don't think we have to look too far to find them.

The very passage that sparked my light bulb moment after chemo points to a deeper purpose behind God allowing trials. Right now, I want to highlight the final part of 1 Peter 1:6-7, which suggests how God can allow suffering, remain good and loving, and even be glorified through it all.

The last time we looked at the passage, I addressed the value of genuine faith. This is what God treasures through our suffering. However, it is through unpacking Peter's metaphor of gold being refined by fire that faith is not merely strengthened when it is refined.

The process of gold being refined by fire is truly remarkable. According to gold experts, here's what happens when gold is refined by fire:

In an exciting process called refining, it is re-liquified in a furnace and then heaped with generous amounts of soda ash and borax. This effectively separates the gold from impurities and other metal traces. There is a range of interesting scientific and technological ways gold can be refined. Whatever the method, what remains is the purest gold on the planet, and it is cast into a beautiful bar that glitters like the sun.

One thing is clear: Gold is not just strengthened through the refining process; it is unmistakably purified. It's transformed into something greater.

So, in line with Peter's metaphor, I believe trials aren't just meant to strengthen our faith; they're meant to transform it. This transformation ties into how God can use trials for a greater purpose while remaining justified in allowing them.

The last part of this passage tells us that it is the proven genuineness, the transformation of our faith, that brings *praise, glory, and honor on the day that Jesus Christ is revealed.*

To some, especially those who question God's existence because of the trials they face, it might seem like God allows people to go through so much just for the sake of transforming their faith. I was in that place at one point, too.

However, I believe God values our faith so much because it's through faith that we are saved and able to have a relationship with Him. When I emphasize faith in life's struggles, I don't mean to suggest that God doesn't care about our physical bodies. He often preserves them through trials, and He chose to do so with mine.

But ultimately, God values our faith because it's what shapes our eternal relationship with Him.

Additionally, the transformation of our faith is part of a bigger purpose that ultimately brings the highest glory to God. When we look at this verse and the rest of Scripture, we see a recurring theme of God's work being the most profound form of transformation. Verses like Romans 8:28 tell us that "in all things God works for the good of those who love him." But how is He able to do this? He redeems us.

Whether it's our faith or any other outcome of a trial, God redeems everything He allows. The word "redeem" is often translated as "to take back," and I can't think of a better way to describe redemption concerning the transformation that trials bring. What the enemy means for evil, God takes back for good. He ultimately transforms our suffering in a way that carries lasting purpose and leads many to Him.

This might seem far-fetched to some. But it's argued that God's ultimate act of redemption was securing our eternal life through Jesus. And if Jesus could redeem our eternity, how could He not redeem a trial that happens within it?

How to Walk Through the Fire

So, now that we've found a purpose for trials, how do we move forward and walk through the fire that God allows to refine us?

This question might be harder than the first. And like before, I don't think I can perfectly guide you through the trial you're facing. However, I have discovered a few things from my own experience in walking through trials that I've found to be helpful.

First and foremost, I would encourage you not to be afraid of asking God "why?" when you encounter a trial. Now, am I saying you should challenge or test God when you can't make sense of it? Of course not! We shouldn't challenge God as if we know better than He does. But I do believe there's a difference between asking God for understanding and questioning Him out of a sense of entitlement.

I find it interesting that some of the most well-known biblical figures didn't shy away from questioning God or asking "why" when they were in tough situations. We see this in Old Testament passages like Psalms 6, 10, and 13. David, the man after God's own heart, starts these Psalms by crying out to God, sometimes questioning Him about the struggles he's facing. In Psalm 13, David even asks, "How long, O Lord? Will you forget me forever? How long will you hide your face from me?" These questions don't come from a place of rebellion. Instead, David is expressing his feeling of God's absence and his confusion about why God seems distant. It seems like he's asking these questions because he genuinely needs God's help.

The questions David asks can be categorized as a lament. Reflecting on biblical laments, Paul E. Miller suggests, "Laments feel disrespectful of God, and yet they are actually faith-filled because they take God seriously." In the examples from Scripture, it's important to note that despite his confusion and frustration, David was still turning to God. His questions came from a place of seeking, not rejecting, God's presence.

This is how I believe it works when we ask God "why" in the face of suffering. We're seeking His help and understanding, wanting to know why something is happening in our lives. Think about a child who's been bullied and asks their parent, "Why was that kid mean to me?" The parent wouldn't accuse the child of being sinful for asking; they would offer comfort and an explanation. In the same way, when we ask God why during a trial, He doesn't condemn us. Instead, He does something even better. He comes to us.

Make no mistake, God doesn't owe us anything! Even in our inability to understand suffering, He is still justified. But when we ask Him "Why?" with the desire to understand, it's a way of genuinely turning to Him. Without a doubt, I believe God responds by meeting us where we are, grabbing our attention, and carrying us forward.

As a result, when we go through trials, we learn to appreciate every day we have. I remember when Mandy reminded me after I broke down hearing that the tumor might be growing, that every day is a gift from God. Even now, being cancer-free for nine years, I'm constantly reminded that tomorrow isn't guaranteed.

One of the best ways I've learned to cultivate appreciation and gratitude is by praising God during pain. It's not that we praise Him for our pain, but we praise Him because He is good despite it. When God brings someone into our lives who wants to pray with us and offer comfort, that's something to praise Him for. When He gives us a moment of peace in the middle of anxiety, that's praiseworthy. When He provides a joyful moment with someone we love, that's also praiseworthy. Ultimately, the fact that God will redeem everything we go through and wipe every tear from our eyes is more than enough reason to offer praise that never stops.

Even so, I recognize that praising God isn't always easy when a tough moment comes. And that brings me to a final piece of advice for walking through trials: We must trust God, even in the hardest moments.

Trusting God is one of those things that's difficult to put into practice. It's defined by being a response to uncertainty. The situations that require us to trust God are often filled with the unknown. We can't see the future, and the instability and insecurity in those moments can be downright terrifying. I've faced that countless times. And, looking back, I wish I'd shown more trust in God when the future was unclear. Yet, I believe God, in His grace, used those moments to teach me how to trust in Him.

One of the best ways I think we can trust in God is by resting on His promises. Taking verses like Jeremiah 29:10-13, Isaiah 41:10, and Philippians 4:6-7 and really meditating on the promises they express can lift our spirits. Doing this strengthens us, both physically and emotionally, and directs our hearts toward trusting God's plans for the next moments we'll face.

In the face of trials, we must trust God. In my trial, He proved that He was always there and that He intended to use every situation to work toward the ultimate healing of my body and the restoration of my faith.

Faith in the Fire

Almost a decade later, I'm still praising God for all He's done through my journey. While life hasn't exactly turned into a cakewalk since finishing treatment, God's provision and faithfulness have never stopped.

God has kept me cancer-free. Through all the follow-up appointments and MRIs, He's protected my brain and even caused it to return to its original shape. Not only have my doctors declared me a cancer survivor, but we're just a couple of years away from them releasing me from follow-up appointments for good.

In His higher ways, God has also guided me through college. Where my doctors had doubts about whether I'd be able to make it, I recently graduated with two degrees. By His grace, God provided the resources and ability to complete a bachelor's in Biblical Studies and a master's in Theological Studies. Strangely enough, I believe God is now calling me to eventually pursue a doctorate.

As amazing as these things are, I believe the greatest evidence of God's faithfulness is in how He's worked through my life. Coming out of the fire and on the other side of cancer, I now have a stronger faith than I've ever had before. All the doubt I was struggling with months earlier has been completely obliterated. Even more, God has called me to pursue vocational ministry. For the rest of my life, I'll dedicate my days to telling people about Jesus's faithfulness and His eternity-saving work.

Do I know every single one of God's plans for the rest of my life? Of course not. Will there be more trials along the way? That seems inevitable. But no matter what life throws my way, I know that God will work through it and faithfully walk with me as I am refined by fire.

www.ingramcontent.com/pod-product-compliance
Lightning Source LLC
Chambersburg PA
CBHW071019280326
41935CB00011B/1409